A Wander in Vetland

by

John Hicks

Table of Contents

For my veterinary colleagues: in memory of "Herriotism" and the noble era of mixed rural practice.

Acknowledgements

This book would never have been written had I not enjoyed such a stimulating time as a farm vet in Southland, New Zealand. To all the players: my veterinary colleagues and staff, the local farmers and pet owners—even those who never knew they participated, and those who never shall, I would like to express my thanks. It has been fun recalling my days with you.

More immediately, I am indebted to Conor Quinn and Norman Bilborough for their encouragement and direction with the manuscript. Also to my wife, Viv, and daughters, Emily and Morwenna: all three have assisted with proof reading and suggestions.

Lastly, I would like to thank Bruce Scott of Regatta Group Publishers for the cover design. It incorporates Sir John Tenniel's famous illustration of the Cheshire Cat from Lewis Carroll's *Alice's Adventures in Wonderland*.

"Curiouser and curiouser!" cried Alice;
"now I'm opening out like the largest telescope that
ever was!..."
– Lewis Carroll, from *Alice's Adventures in*
Wonderland.

Every veterinary practitioner presented with a patient knows that successful treatment depends on an accurate diagnosis. One of the key steps involves extracting a *clinical history* from the owner: When did the symptoms first appear? What did you notice? How frequently is this recurring? At the same time a subjective assessment has to be made about the reliability of the information received. The owners may not realise the importance of this process; but if you are the vet, it's up to you to find out. Your patient cannot tell you what happened, but the owner often can. Your patient cannot lie, but his owner sometimes will: he may wish to conceal that "Zac" is acting strangely because he has been fed cannabis cookies; that "Rust" is stiff and sore because of the lead pellets in his back from a careless shot; or omit to mention the stone he threw at "Teak" to stop him barking. A good clinician needs to be a detective. He needs to be curious. It becomes an ingrained habit.

I confess to a curiosity about the history of medicine and surgery. It is probably driven by the personal gratitude I feel to have lived in an era when medicine has been practised with rationality and humanity. It is a matter of lucky timing—by a mere hundred and fifty years or so—that I have evaded the abominable barbarities of the past. I found that the more

I dug into the mire of medical history, the more my idle curiosity turned into a grim fascination.

This interest has led me to link the curiosities I discovered to my experiences in modern veterinary practice. I admit to a certain randomness in this approach, and I lay no claim to balance. To my mind a description of Neolithic trephination techniques sits neatly beside a consideration of more modern methods of drilling holes in skulls; and any account of hemlock poisoning would be incomplete without going back to 399 BC, the year of Socrates' death. Bladder stones in cats and dogs inevitably invite comparison with Samuel Pepys' famous affliction; and how could I not avoid straying into the use of goose quills by eunuchs? St. Blaise, is the foremost veterinary saint and his cruel death must surely rate inclusion in any historical study of the veterinary profession.

We have all been shaped by history, so I have also included personal curiosities linking members of my family to cannibalism and the murder of a missionary in New Zealand, and to the St Bartholomew Massacre in France.

But there is an inbuilt distortion: history compresses time. Thousands of years can be dispensed in a single paragraph; whereas the present is lived in real time. We must compensate for this if we are to learn from history, otherwise we fail to recognise the significance of the changes occurring in our own lifetimes until it is too late: until they, too, have been consigned to history.

This is certainly true of the veterinary profession, which is presently undergoing a period of dramatic re-adjustment, just as it did a hundred years ago with the demise of the working horse. In an overpopulated world clamouring for food, pastoral farming is moving towards the vast scale and efficiencies we have seen in the pig and poultry industries over the last few decades: factory farming. For this and other reasons farm animal practice, as so lovingly depicted by James Herriot, is disappearing. I feel lucky to have been part of a proud tradition and do not envy today's farm vets the less colourful future to which they seem destined.

Unfortunately for the modern teller of veterinary tales, the tough, idiosyncratic characters on whom James Herriot drew so deeply, are a vanishing breed. It is no longer enough for farmers to be honest toilers. To be successful, they now need to be well-educated businessmen. Their vets have changed with them. I have tried to give some realistic perspectives of life as a vet during my times, but a lot of what I have written is an indulgence: a concentration of the truly remarkable or amusing incidents that crop up all too rarely in a profession that increasingly consigns its participants to desk work and cerebral pursuits behind a computer screen.

A Wander in Vetland was compiled during a period of major change in my life. I was recovering from some sobering adventures with cancer, and had recently retired from the profession that had given me many enjoyable years. This book is a tribute to those years, and to the people with whom I shared a working life full of challenges, much laughter, and not a few trials.

I shall begin in the middle. 1865 seems as good a time as any in which to start my wander. It was the year that Lewis Carroll wrote *Alice's Adventures in Wonderland*, but on the other side of the world something much more sinister was going on...

Chapter One

Kereopa and Emma Lanfear's Husband

And thine eye shall not pity; but life shall go for life,
eye for eye, tooth for tooth, hand for hand, foot for foot.
Deuteronomy 19:21

When Viv and I decided I should accept a veterinary
position in New Zealand, some of my fellow students
were aghast. One of the more image conscious ones—
he made a point of driving around with a riding hat and
crop prominently displayed on the rear shelf of his car
—was aghast. "You can't be serious! The women over
there still run around in print frocks." Another wag
added that the Maoris wore grass skirts and still
practised cannibalism. His information was about 140
years out of date but, if anything, it did more to pique
our curiosity than to deter us in our adventure.
However, in a strange way, he was not as far off the
mark as might be imagined. When I married Vivien
Lanfear I had no knowledge of any New Zealand ghosts
in her past; neither had she. It wasn't until many years
later that Viv's mother, while researching family
history, discovered the Lanfears' tenuous link to
nineteenth century New Zealand.

~

Emma Volkner (née Martha Emma Lanfear), was safely
in Auckland while Kereopa te Rau—ignoble savage—
was choking on her husband's eyes. Carl Volkner's
death was one among many bookmarks in the

8

upheavals of the young colony during the New Zealand Wars, but its manner evokes such fearsome imagery that cautious modern historians, after the elapse of nearly 150 years, avoid the details—perhaps for fear of stirring racial prejudices.

Until his death Volkner had lived for four years as a missionary among the Maori at Opotiki, on the East Coast of the North Island. He was working for the Church Missionary Society under the redoubtable Bishop Selwyn. Unfortunately, it was also suspected by some Maori that Volkner was a government spy.

In February 1865 the *Hauhaus*, a breakaway group of *Pai Marire*, descended on Volkner's settlement at Opotiki. Pai Marire, was a new, Maori version of Christianity. Literally translated its name means "The Good and the Peaceful". The Hauhaus were radicals within it, and they were anything but good or peaceful.

Volkner and his wife were in Auckland at the time of the raid, obtaining medicines for a typhoid epidemic at the mission. While there, Volkner received a letter from the rebels ordering him not to return to Opotiki. Victorian missionaries were made of stern stuff and he could not be dissuaded from carrying out what he saw as his duty. Leaving Emma in Auckland for safety, he returned to his mission on 1st March to find it ransacked, and the contents of his house sold. He was held captive by the Hauhaus and condemned to death by Kereopa, their leader. In doing this he was disobeying the orders of Te Ua, his own leader. But Kereopa was headstrong and had become carried away by the power he wielded over his followers, and those of Volkner's parishioners whom he had managed to convert.

On the 2nd March 1865, Volkner was marched into his church by an armed guard. Kereopa stripped him of his coat and waistcoat and dressed in them himself. He then ordered the execution. Volkner was led outside and, after kneeling to pray and saying farewell to some of his parishioners, he was hung from a large willow tree.

He was hauled up and down, shot at a few times and left hanging for about an hour, and then his body was lowered and decapitated with an axe. Kereopa took the communion chalice from the church vestry and filled it with blood—"as it spouted forth"—by one account. [An over-imaginative exaggeration, unless Volkner were still alive: blood only spouts when the heart is pumping.] Kereopa then took the chalice and Volkner's head and led his people back into the church.

What follows is not for the squeamish. Even those of us fed a steady diet of Grimm's fairy tales in our childhoods may not be prepared for the bit about the eyes. Some have phobias about eyes as acute as any about spiders or snakes. I was always surprised when I encountered such people in my veterinary career: they would no more contemplate putting drops into eyes of their pet dog, than you or I would volunteer to clean the teeth of a crocodile.

Kereopa did not share these fears. He stood on the pulpit and, placing Volkner's head on the lectern he gouged out both eyes, supposedly with his fingers. He held up an eye in each hand between finger and thumb and, proclaiming that one was the parliament of England, and the other the law of New Zealand, he swallowed them, one after the other. The second eye, purportedly, stuck in his throat and he "called" [surely beckoned] for a drink of water to help him swallow it. At this stage Volkner's head dropped to the floor and Kereopa picked it up, re-setting the eyeless, bloody head in front of him on the lectern.

The written accounts of the day summon to mind a scene of demonic savagery: Kereopa, in Volkner's long black coat, hypnotically steering his congregation of fearful converts towards the cannibalism of their recent pasts.

The communion chalice was passed around. Those who drank the blood were persuaded that they would obtain knowledge of the English tongue and be able to work miracles. This would not have been an alien concept to them: by eating a vanquished enemy you absorbed his mana. Cannibalism was widely practised by Maori in the aftermath of inter-tribal warfare until well into the 1830s. So it is not surprising that although many were astounded by the killing of a missionary who had been with them for so long, and some tried to prevent it; they were powerless before Kereopa and his armed men, and feared his god and his magic incantations.

While Kereopa may have stirred the primal sensibilities of some of his people, he was politically inept. The outrage he caused by this incident, and another murder that he committed soon afterwards, was used by the government and ministers to make successful representations to the Secretary of State to retain Imperial troops in New Zealand. He was captured and executed in 1872. Opotiki was declared a military settlement and units of Armed Constabulary were stationed there for several years.

Emma's father, and Viv's ancestor, the Reverend William Lanfear of the village of Christian Malford in Wiltshire, died in 1875. Twelve thousand miles separated him from the awful tragedy of his son-in-law's death and many months must have elapsed before he heard from his daughter.

Emma had married late, at the age of forty-four. After eleven years of marriage to Carl Volkner there were no children. Her genteel early upbringing as the daughter of a country vicar would have borne many similarities to that of another much more famous vicar's daughter: Jane Austen. The two were raised in the same corner of England and only a few years separated them, so the genteel lifestyles depicted in Jane Austen's peerless prose could be a useful guide to the life Emma Lanfear may have known. It is hard to imagine how this would have equipped her for her later life. Was she an adventurous woman to whom life in the colonies presented an irresistible opportunity? Or was she reluctantly drawn by her love for a man, of undoubted principle and religious conviction, into this horrific situation?

My research leads me to believe that neither of these views is correct. I had envisioned a bereft fifty-five year old widow alone in a small town at the furthest extremity of civilisation, with no emotional support and struggling to cope with the ghastly news as best she could. But in this view I was guilty of ignoring the emotional conditioning which made these nineteenth century missionaries what they were. Emma, it seems, was imbued with more than enough faith to guide her through her loss. *The New Zealand Church Gazette* records that the "crushing blow", broken to her by Bishop Selwyn, was borne with "meek submission" and that she prayed for her husband's murderers. It claimed that she found comfort in the thought that "the blood of the martyrs is the seed of the church". Another account (*Church and People*) records that she received the news "with true Christian courage, saying only, 'So he has won the crown'".

In January 1866 Emma Lanfear returned to England and made her home with her brother and his family, "finding true consolation in her widowed life by living only for others". She died on 27th January 1878. According to her sisters-in-law her last intelligible words were "I am almost come home" and, finally "I know that I am perfect in Christ, nothing can avail me, and I have perfect peace in Him". She then sank back on her pillow and died. "Her death was like her life, full of light and peace." No doubt she lies at rest in some corner of a country churchyard, in the land of her birth.

Carl Volkner's headless body was buried behind the church that he built at Opotiki, soon to be sanctified as the Church of St. Stephen the Martyr. When the church was extended in 1910 his grave came within the Sanctuary. His head suffered a different fate. It was smoked for preservation and carried off for use in Hauhau rituals. Its final resting place is not known.

~

Kereopa's performance is memorable for all the wrong reasons. The tissues binding the eye into its socket are tough. Gouging out Volkner's eyes bare-handedly was no mean feat. It would have been a gruesome struggle, with one hand gripping the awkward and slippery head, while the fingernails of the other tore through the conjunctival membranes to reach behind the eyeball. Perhaps, given the setting, there has been a bit of subliminal scriptural interpolation here: *...And if thine eye offend thee, pluck it out and cast it from thee...* There: it's easy! These days women pluck their eyebrows, but obviously, in biblical times, people were more inclined to go the whole hog.

We can also deduce that Kereopa must have had a very big mouth. The visible part of the eye is only a fraction of the surface of the eyeball. In fact, the human eye has a diameter of roughly four centimetres, which is only marginally less than that of a golf ball. If you imagined Kereopa popping these eyes into his mouth—like we, as children, popped in those old fashioned sweets we knew as "gobstoppers"—and swallowing them in one gulp, think again. The sclera, the white covering of the eyeball, is very tough and elastic. These eyes would have required chewing before swallowing: the moment when *grisly*, acquires teeth and becomes *gristly*. So although the eyewitness descriptions lead readers to imagine a theatrical "pop and swallow"; the reality could have been even more gruesome if, in fact, it occurred as described. No wonder he called for a glass of water.

The medically minded will be aware that Kereopa's unrestrained eating habits exposed him to considerable risks. There was, as we have mentioned, a typhoid epidemic in Opotiki at the time, and cannibalism exposes its participants to extreme risk from hepatitis and many other diseases, although Maori generally mitigated this by cooking. However, even cooking will not destroy prions. These are the agents responsible for Scrapie in sheep and "Mad Cow Disease" (Bovine Spongiform Encephalopathy, BSE) in cattle. BSE was caused by adding Scrapie infected sheep meat to cattle rations. Likewise, prions and cannibalism have been linked in humans. The South Foré people of New Guinea unwittingly infected themselves with Kuru, a prion disease, by eating the brains of their dead relatives. Kuru caused emaciation and contracted face muscles and was known by the South Foré as "laughing sickness". Kereopa would have been unaware of this particular disease. It would be another century before its cause was unravelled.

Kereopa committed a horrendous crime, but as to the details, how much is truth, how much polemic? There is no doubt that political mileage was gained for the settlers by maximising the horror of the event; but it has to be acknowledged that atrocities were committed by both sides in this vicious, guerrilla stage of the Maori Wars. The colonial forces with their Maori allies (there being Maori fighting on both sides) took no prisoners, gave no quarter and looted, killed, and burnt villages and destroyed crops.

On the other hand, omission of the details from modern history books smacks of political correctness. Some well respected general histories of New Zealand cover the whole episode in less than one sentence: "Kereopa Te Rau…was involved in the killing of the missionary Carl Volkner…" or, from The Oxford History of New Zealand (1992): "Yet, for all this, it was the murder of the missionary Carl Sylvius Volkner at Opotiki and Te Kooti's massacre of thirty-three settlers and thirty-seven kupapa ('friendly') Maori at Poverty Bay in 1868 that left the most enduring memories." This is scant treatment of such a dramatic episode in New Zealand history in an otherwise detailed and lengthy book.

We need to rake up such ghosts from the past because human nature in the raw—around the world— has led us to plumb depths we all must acknowledge, the better to avoid their repetition. Those of us with European ancestry cannot afford to gloat on our supposedly superior civilisation. Our histories are frighteningly replete with secular and religious savagery, and the fate of Viv's saintly antecedent pales into insignificance beside the persecution experienced by my mother's ancestors.

Chapter Two

The Roots of Prejudice

God seems to have forgotten all I have done for him.
Louis XIV

The influence of history has a long reach. Kereopa's crime played no part in Viv's formative years, but the calamitous persecution of my ancestors in France— several centuries before Kereopa was born—certainly influenced mine, and today there are millions around the world who could claim common cause with me.

The French kings in the sixteenth century, according to Nancy Mitford, were regarded—indeed, regarded themselves—as "Viceroys of the Almighty". France was a Roman Catholic theocracy and Roman Catholicism was compulsory. This fusion of church and state existed before the reign of Louis XIV the "Sun King" (1643 – 1715), although his glittering decadence exemplified some of the worst aspects of absolute power. Whenever he worshipped God in his chapel, his courtiers—with their backs to the altar—faced their king and worshipped him.

There were bound to be dissidents unable to tolerate life as the subjects of the licentious and unjust monarchs who claimed divine authority over them. A Protestant reformation swept through France in the early fifteenth century. They believed in salvation through individual faith and the right of individuals to interpret the scriptures for themselves without the need for intercession by the state, or even a church hierarchy. But the government would not tolerate such freedom of

17

thought. In 1536 it issued a general edict that encouraged the extermination of Protestants.

Despite this, or because of it, French Protestantism continued to grow. The Huguenots, as they came to be known, were in increasing conflict with the authorities. In 1562, twelve hundred Huguenots were slain at Vassey. This ignited the French Wars of Religion which devastated France for the next thirty-five years. The worst atrocity was the St Bartholomew Massacre of 1572, instigated on the orders of Charles IX. Over three bloody days, more than eight thousand Huguenots were murdered in Paris alone. Many had their throats slashed by Swiss mercenaries, the king's guards, or his "noble" allies, the Duke of Guise and his followers. If we consider that the human body contains around five litres (just over a gallon) of blood, the jolting reality of this slaughter would have been thousands of gallons of it splashing onto cobbled streets, spraying onto walls and soaking into furnishings. Accounts of atrocities often resort to clichés about "rivers of blood"; in this case the description is probably warranted.

The massacres spread throughout the country.

How easy it is to overlook the suffering, the stench and the flies, in the dry pages of history books. The river Rhone was choked with corpses from the massacre in Lyons and the citizens of Arles were unable to drink its water for three months. In the valley of the Loire, wolves came down from the hills to feast on the decaying bodies.

When the news reached Rome, Pope Gregory XIII was jubilant. He made several moves that were unlikely to endear him, or his office, to any remaining Protestants. He oversaw a procession of thanksgiving in Rome, and thanked God in prayer for having "granted the Catholic people a glorious triumph over a perfidious race". The artist Vasari was commissioned to paint scenes of the triumph of "The Most Christian King" over the Huguenots in one of the Vatican apartments. A commemorative medal was struck, featuring corpses of the slain on the "tails" side. This behaviour by the head of the Roman Catholic Church—believed by its adherents to be God's infallible representative on earth—explains why there would never be reconciliation between the two faiths.

The persecution ended in 1598 when Henry IV, himself a Huguenot, signed the Edict of Nantes. At last Huguenots were permitted to practice their faith, but only in twenty specified "free" cities. However, when Henry IV was assassinated by a Catholic fanatic in 1610, the persecution resumed. The free cities gradually fell to the forces of Cardinal Richelieu, and "Sun King" Louis XIV revoked the Edict of Nantes in 1685. Huguenots were tortured, burnt at the stake or, if they were able-bodied, condemned to a miserable and short life as galley slaves. The French navy increased its galleys from six to forty. Each employed two hundred slaves, and Huguenots found themselves rowing alongside criminals and Turks captured in the Barbary wars. Huguenot churches and houses were destroyed. Huguenot children were forcibly removed from their parents and educated by Roman Catholic monks or nuns. Mixed marriages were forbidden and the children of existing ones declared illegitimate. When Protestants became ill they were taken to state hospitals so that their last moments could be supervised by a priest. In the wealthy towns of southern France, where Protestantism thrived, a policy named *Dragonnades* was imposed—regiments of ill-disciplined dragoons were compulsorily billeted in Protestant households where they had licence to create havoc. Under Louvois,

Louis XIV's war minister, rape and plunder went unpunished. The soldiers were encouraged to mistreat their unfortunate hosts in every way possible. Murder and torture became commonplace.

The net was tightened: emigration was declared illegal. Nevertheless, by various estimates between two hundred and fifty and four hundred thousand Huguenots fled to other European countries, South Africa and North America. An equal number were killed in France itself. Many of these were affluent trades' people, artisans and skilled workers that France could ill-afford to lose. The persecution of the Huguenots, aside from being morally repugnant, was economically disastrous for France. An Edict of Toleration in 1787 partially restored the rights of French Huguenots, and their church was fully legalised in 1802.

It was a rather late move. By this time forty thousand Huguenots had settled in Britain, where their skills were welcomed. Among them were my mother's ancestors, the Dorées, who came to London. They were originally silk-weavers. One of their descendants, George Dorée, supplied the velvet for Edward VII's coronation robes in 1901. It is no surprise that the Huguenots brought with them a total contempt for papacy, and anything connected with the Church of Rome. My own mother, bless her, inherited a full complement of this baggage. Most of her family members that I knew, as a child, could be described as rabidly anti-Catholic. Mum's animosity was not personal, but directed towards the institution itself.

It was also from her French ancestors, I assume, that Mum derived her Latin temperament, and a tendency to scandalous exaggeration. The latter was an idiosyncrasy that I found confusing, as a child. Are men with jug-handle ears invariably poor drivers? What is so dangerous about liver-lipped politicians? But children love drama and eccentricity, and Mum's hyperbole was couched in such wonderfully colourful language; how could we resist? Small wonder that my brother and I sometimes held confused perspectives. How were we to know that many of her pronouncements on topics, such as burning the Pope, were outrageous rhetoric?— especially when a guiding principle of Mum's life was to treat all she met with kindness. In spite of her diatribes against their faith, some of her best friends were Catholics! When, as a youngster, I met them I was surprised that their teeth had not been worn down from "chewing the pews" of their local church—an occupation which, my mother had mistakenly led me to believe, occupied "all their waking hours". Later I was to learn that this strange expression was a linguistic anomaly—one of many family eccentricities—a term of derision applying to anyone of overly religious persuasion.

It would be a mistake to assume that Protestants would have been models of tolerance had the boot been on the other foot. Burning at the stake was not solely an atrocity inflicted by Roman Catholics on Protestants. Conflicting protestant sects—Lutherans, Calvinists, Anabaptists, Deists, Unitarianists—denounced each other for perceived heresy and contrived punishments every bit as shocking as those of the Roman Catholic Inquisition, although never on the same scale. They burnt and hanged each other, and some designed even more bizarre fates for those who dared to believe differently.

The Anabaptists practised adult baptism by total immersion in water. It seems innocuous enough to us, but sixteenth century Lutherans in the state of Zurich thought otherwise. They inflicted prolonged total immersion in water—death by drowning—on any Anabaptists they managed to entrap.

Our ancestors were an intolerant lot.

~

It was my mother's fate to marry a Liverpudlian. He was, as you might expect, not a Roman Catholic, but she was now destined to live in Liverpool, the most Catholic of British cities. During my childhood, the first Roman Catholic cathedral to be built on English soil since the Reformation, was erected in Liverpool. It is an unconventional and strikingly modern concrete-and-glass structure, with a cylindrical tower soaring over its conical base. The Mersey Tunnel, connecting Liverpool with the Wirral peninsula on the other side of the Mersey is, to Liverpudlians, an iconic landmark. In their inimitable way, they soon dubbed their new cathedral the "Mersey Funnel".

Our house in Liverpool was a large Victorian semi-detached. There was a polished mahogany banister from the top floor, and my brother and I could sit astride it and slide down all four-stories, much to the envy of visiting children who came from modern, less characterful homes. There was also a damp and spooky cellar that an imaginative child could only dread. After I discovered the vivid horror stories of Edgar Allan Poe, my visits there to bring up buckets of coal for my parents, became personal struggles—the terror of which I failed to impart to them. "Don't be so damn silly!" was their pragmatic response, and I knew the truth of their words. But I was like a moth to a flame; I found it hard to resist any author of the macabre. WW Jacobs, Bram Stoker and Dennis Wheatley frizzled the flight path of my tender soul. We all thrive on a bit of fear: bouts of terror add piquancy to life.

Beyond the high and sooty brick wall of our back garden arose a large neo-gothic structure, its sandstone masonry blackened by pollution. Its steep slate roof climbed forever, towards the leaden skies. This was the local Catholic church.

With a catapult it was possible to skim pebbles up this roof, much as one skips flat pebbles across a calm pond. The angles were more challenging but, if you if got it right, those stones would bounce with alluring pitch variation (and I am referring to tonal quality here) nearly to the apex of the roof and then, losing all impetus, roll lazily down—gathering pace as they thudded into the gutter. Marbles were the best, but youthful penury precluded their frequent use.

The amazing thing about all this was that Mum turned a blind eye to my brother's and my delinquency. Yes! Our mother! Our mother who usually came down hard on anything less than impeccable behaviour. Little did we realise that we, like her, were mere pawns in an ancient game—exacting vengeance for the St Bartholomew Massacre and all the other atrocities the Roman Catholics had inflicted on innocent Protestants over previous centuries. And so, with this outlet for the devil in us, we periodically plied that roof with pebbles. If the pinging resonance of the hard stones on those slates was obvious to us, what acoustic embellishment did it provide for those at worship within? We were soon to find out.

The priest came knocking on our door. My mother dealt with him courteously, and he was permitted to have a word in private with my brother and me. This was, perhaps, my first encounter with a representative of the Roman Catholic faith. He was a gentle young man. He appealed to our better natures and encouraged us to desist from interrupting his services. We were impressed. We desisted.

~

Beneath my mother's English veneer, her Latin temperament flared. This, magnified by her Gallic gift for hyperbole, spared us any perception of the mundane. She fiercely loved the birds in her garden— our small oasis of green set in its brick and concrete surrounds. No winter passed without food for the blue tits, blackbirds, thrushes or anything else able to survive the depredations of the cats besieging us. Meg, our Fox Terrier cross, was programmed to keep the coast clear of cats, many of which were encouraged by the priest's housekeeper's habit of laying out regular fish left-overs on the seminary steps—next to the church. The whole neighbourhood, my mother insisted, was "snowing with millions of stray cats". And "that trollop" who was "living with the priest" set up an orgy of feasting for them every Friday evening.

Meg picked up on these vibes and would become frantic if she saw any cats in her territory. She responded to the word "cats", as any normal dog responds to the word "walk"; but we could induce her to even greater hysteria with a cry of "coggers' moggies". Frantically she'd lurch for the back door, her legs a blur of useless energy scrabbling for purchase on the slippery tiles. Suddenly she would gain traction, find voice, and shoot outside like a cork from a bottle. Her banshee screams reached a crescendo as she locked on to her quarry, yet in her long life she contrived never to catch a single cat. They had plenty of warning, and she wasn't stupid. If they stood their ground and didn't run, she pretended she couldn't see them.

"Cogger" is a Liverpudlian term for Roman Catholic. In the main, Liverpudlians are a tolerant lot, and I don't believe that the word is used derogatively. In Liverpool's polluted past I can only surmise it was the closest approximation its citizens could make to the correct pronunciation through their phlegm-clogged nasal passages.

Honesty compels me to continue with my story, though as a vet of some longstanding, it is with the utmost reluctance that I proceed from this point …

My brother and I were enlisted in the war against cats. Armed with those same catapults that propelled missiles up the church roof, Mum encouraged us to repel any cats that had the audacity to parade in our garden, especially those with the cheek to sit next to her bird feeders waiting to trap a feathered snack or plaything.

From our third or fourth floor windows we had a wonderful range of fire. A pebble sizzling into the vegetation beside an unsuspecting cat merely arouses its curiosity. It assumes there is another mouse rustling about for it to torture. You can take three or four pots at a naïve cat: one that has not been caught out before. And then, a strike! A thud, a yowl, a frantic scramble, and over the wall she goes! Cats have good memories and we kept our garden relatively clear in this manner.

The moral of this tale is that our attitude to animals, as to people of other religious persuasions, is a learned response. We can be conditioned to persecute without remorse and we are inconsistent in our application of moral standards. Rats are rewarding pets, yet I would have no fear of retribution from outraged rat owners if I had just described a teenage rat-hunting expedition; but this catapult confession has the potential to expose me to the vitriol of every cat owning member of the public. Many would regard my behaviour as "beyond the pale". The point is that I was programmed to be a dog lover and a cat hater. Seeds of prejudice, sown early, readily take root.

Other cultures raise their children to despise dogs. The only human contact a dog is likely to receive in many Arab countries is a violent one, from a foot or stone: all in the name of religion. Yet other religious philosophies revere all forms of life, even those lowlier than rats.

Who decides where to site the pale beyond which we must not stray? In the past, religious faiths have determined our moral boundaries, but the sufferings of my Huguenot ancestors at the dictates of men of unbounded religiosity inclines me to favour an education system that enables us to be humble and appreciate that we are not at the apex of creation, but a mere part of it; and that of all the creatures on this planet we are, probably, the most intelligent and, almost certainly, the least perfect—because we should know better.

Chapter Three

Feckless in Ireland

It ain't the parts of the Bible that I can't understand that bother me, it is the parts that I do understand – Mark Twain

Sunday Chapel, at a Liverpool college for boarding school boys, 1965

I believe in God the Father Almighty, Maker of Heaven and earth. And in Jesus Christ his only Son, our Lord; who was conceived by the Holy Ghost, Born of the Virgin Mary, Suffered under Pontius Pilate, Was crucified, dead, and buried, He descended into hell; The third day he rose again from the dead, He ascended into heaven, And sitteth on the right hand of God the Father Almighty; From whence he shall come to judge the quick and the dead.

Once again I found the familiar words tumbling out of my mouth, indeed, they seemed to be tumbling out of the mouths of everyone except for the new boy on my right—stumbling would be a better way to describe his effort. Of course Brown had only started boarding that term and had yet to learn the Apostles' Creed off pat. Regular attendance at chapel would soon sort that out. Some of the other boys sniggered smugly. We believed in all sorts of things that Brown evidently didn't. We believed in: *the Holy Ghost; The holy Catholick Church; The Communion of Saints; The forgiveness of sins; The Resurrection of the body, And the Life everlasting. Amen.* And really! That *aymen* from Brown was a dead giveaway. We all knew it should be *ahmen.* You couldn't cheat by reading it from the *Book of Common Prayer*—not that it would have

27

been easy from its dense print of lurching capitals and idiosyncratic punctuation. Oh no! You had to speak it from the heart! It was important to inflect the words properly ... to pause in the right places. Those who rushed on when the rest had stopped found themselves in a very exposed position. Religious etiquette was a minefield. You could betray your ignorance in so many ways, like when you didn't sink to your knees at one with the rest of the congregation, or emulate their postures of sombre reflection as, with bowed heads and piously closed eyes, they joined in the Reverend Black's incantations—though who would notice such transgressions was a matter for cynical conjecture. Out of the corner of my eye I could see that Brown was catching on quickly.

There were lots of questions. Earlier in my childhood I had wondered if Pontius Pilate drove his tugboat around the Sea of Galilee like Clive Digby's dad, who was a pilot on the river Mersey. Was *a communion of saints* a collective noun: as prosaic as *a flock of sheep*, as alliterative as *a gaggle of geese*, as uplifting as *an exaltation of larks*, as ridiculous as an *observance of hermits* or as sinister as *a coven of witches*? Why did we believe in the holy *Catholick* Church when we were supposed to be Anglicans? And how could Mary have let a ghost, holy or secular, anywhere near her? When I was much older I learned that He had, in fact, impregnated Mary another way: not down below; for there was nothing dirty or sinful about this conception. No! He had waxed (and, no doubt, waned) in her ear—which one, or both, is not clear. Nuns wore wimples covering the sides of their heads in modest acknowledgement of this miracle, lest the sight of even these innocent orifices could lead the thoughts of mortal men towards the sin of copulation.

Church sermons are fertile breeding grounds for lateral thinkers.

It brought to my mind the vision of a man trying to squirm through the eye of a needle. Perhaps I had mixed my metaphors. How did it go? Yes… *for it is easier for a camel to go through the eye of a needle than for a rich man to enter the Kingdom of Heaven.*

The Reverend Black posed elegantly in his chasuble as he delivered his sermon and led us in the Lord's Prayer. Somehow, I doubted he would trade in his Rover for a bicycle and conduct his next sermon in sackcloth. Such doubts, rather formless in my youthful teens, but moulded here by life's experiences, continued:

And lead us not into temptation. Even though you've swamped our bodies with testosterone, told us that fornication is a sin, and advocated chastity before marriage? We are to be tempted for many years before we may, with the blessing of the church, indulge our sinful appetites. Meanwhile your messenger will preach us an impossible message of self-control.

As we forgive them that trespass against us. Except for Makliski—abandoned to the boarding school by his recently divorced parents. We didn't forgive him for carving "The Kinks" into one of our pews. We expelled him, didn't we?

I wasn't good enough to be a Christian, but neither, I strongly suspected, was the Reverend who stood proudly before us. And so it came to pass that I chose not to be confirmed when Brown, along with many others of my peers, claimed that they did, truly, believe and knew that the wine they drank at communion was Christ's blood. This was the full Monty: Anglo-Catholic high-church transubstantiation. Yet I couldn't even believe in the Lutheran cop-out, consubstantiation:

that the blood and flesh of Christ merely coexisted with the wine and bread consumed at the Eucharist.

But thank you, Reverend, for the insights you gave me in my early youth. Life promised to be a delicious paradox from which, to extract maximum enjoyment, I needed to develop a strong sense of irony. I accepted that many good Christians have led exemplary lives—excellent life models for the rest of us to follow—and that organised religion has inspired great architecture, wonderful music and, through the King James Bible, developed the poetry of our language. Yet, in spite of all this, absolute faith still evades me. I remain a heretic—free to choose what I believe—and further, the calumnies committed in the name of religion convince me that blind faith is a menace to society. It is the duty of everyone to question and to choose for themselves.

~

The Emerald Isle would not normally be regarded as a hallowed destination for the youth of one of England's staunchly Church of England public schools. But if that school happened to be in Liverpool, at least you could say that it was convenient. It was easy enough to hop on the ferry and swap the stench of the Mersey for the sniffy Liffey. So, one summer holiday, in the early 1960s, Ireland became the destination of a troop of about twenty Boy Scouts from my school. We set out to visit the lair of the "bog-Irish" Roman Catholics—as my mother would have it—the home of those idle navvies who "breast fed their shovels" beside every road works in Liverpool. Couched in such overblown terms, I felt like Jonathan Swift's Gulliver about to embark on one of his exotic travels. And perhaps I was not so far off the mark, for Jonathan Swift, born in

Dublin, remains one of the many brilliant literary stars of Ireland, and a he was a sarcastic bastard into the bargain.

Beyond Dublin, the country was green—yes, emerald—and well wooded. We were heading for the Wicklow Mountains. Eire had a special feel, all its own. We had stepped back in time. Callow as I was, in my tender early teens, I had little idea of the organisation that went into making arrangements for a scout camp, but those responsible had chosen well. We set up our bell tents in a sheltered meadow. We were surrounded on three sides by trees, handy to running water and wood for our fires. One of the first tasks was to erect a flagpole. Over the days we constructed towers and bridges from spars and ropes, learned about lashings and knots, campfires and billies, kit inspections and night hikes, played rounders with tennis balls and, when no adult was looking, chicken with sheath knives—the whole boy scout experience.

Each morning started with prayers under the flag, and every evening ended with a singsong round the campfire. I hated the conformity of both of these extremes; no matter how pissed off with life you might have felt—and, believe me, sometimes teenagers do succumb to vague feelings of negativity—*Ging gang goolie, goolie, goolie, goolie watcha* or *I'm riding along on the crest of a wave* was the tonic for you! Thank you very much Robert Baden Powell.

The flag was a serious part of our ritual. The Union Jack has to be folded correctly. Is the broad, diagonal stripe at the top or bottom? Never let it touch the ground. When does the patrol leader salute? Then the morning prayers: the Union Jack and C of E flaunted in holy alliance. Our flag was launched aloft and proudly unfurled over the verdant pastures of Ireland. It blessed the rising voices of the little Anglicans circled beneath its protection. I'm sure it was all done in unthinking innocence, but obviously that was not the way some of the locals saw it. One morning our flagpole wasn't there. It wasn't a hatchet job: nothing as dramatic as Hone Heke's efforts to destroy this symbol of British sovereignty at Kororareka. Our pole and its supporting guys were neatly stowed—an elegant yet forceful statement by locals unknown, rather than an act of vandalism.

Displays of the Union Jack were abandoned for the rest of our camp. Quite possibly the flag itself had been "confiscated". It was a point well made. In addition, we were no longer to wear our scout uniforms at the camp. From now on it was strictly mufti—so woggles, lanyards and neckerchiefs were out; but the true reason was never leaked to us. We may have been politically naïve, but the letters I, R and A were not unknown to us. Boys being boys, there were all sorts of rumours about Mr B, our scoutmaster, sleeping with a shotgun under his camp bed. It would have been a great opportunity to have given us a balanced lesson in Irish history, but as you would expect, anything we had been taught at that stage came with a distinctly Cromwellian slant. It wasn't till years later, after living in New Zealand, that I gained a more mature understanding, from a colonial viewpoint, of cultural imperialism.

Two other episodes remain imprinted on my mind from that holiday. One involved a middle-aged woman rushing out of her cottage at the end of a remote valley to speak to us, a patrol of six Boy Scouts, solely because we were Protestants. Hers was the only Protestant family in the district. We gratefully consumed the proffered refreshments and, tired and hungry boys that we were, thought no more of it. On reflection, it seems that there is more solace to be gained from religion for those who worship in the same manner as their neighbours. Organised religion, of no matter what denomination, does not reward individuality.

Very early one morning we returned by coach to Dublin, travelling in full Boy Scout regalia. Weary and hungry, we traipsed the streets down towards the quay and our boat. To our joy, someone found a bright and cheerful breakfast bar. A jovial Dubliner gestured us inside and we sat side-by-side on the tall stools and slavered over the choices of full cooked breakfasts. I was the last one in and sat at the end of the row of hungry boys. The seat next to me was almost immediately occupied by a very unsteady and untidily attired woman. She had evidently been eating eggs and bacon because, as she tried to engage me in conversation, a hail of yolk chunks showered from her mouth. "You focking English pig". It was an interesting, but not very encouraging, opening gambit. I had not had a wide experience of drunks before, but I was beginning to suspect that this lady was over the limit. Her slurred diction was not conducive to effective communication, so I concentrated—as unobtrusively and politely as possible—on shielding my bacon and eggs from the gathering garnish of labial detritus. Besides, I was a bit thrown by the transposed vowel in that unutterable second word. We didn't say it like that. Boy Scouts are not saints; we used the "f" word whenever we judged we were not in danger of being overheard by adults—for it was certainly a flogging offence—but this "lady" seemed to have transposed the central vowel. I would get confirmation of this in due course.

In the face of such unexpected aggression I went into autopilot and tried to shut her out of my mind. Ignoring her, however, didn't help. If anything she was working herself into an even greater frenzy. What should I do? We were always taught to be polite to ladies and so, in the face of her insistence I made the mistake of asking, "I'm sorry, what did you say?"

"You heard me, you focking English pig." Yes, I was callow and tender. I had not been exposed to naked hatred from a total stranger, drunken or otherwise, at such close quarters. And this screaming harridan meant business. She took off her stiletto shoe and raised it above her head. Before she could bring it down on me, a hand grabbed her wrist from behind and, still screaming and swearing, she was shepherded onto the street by the firm but gentle hand of the proprietor. Our genial host had rescued me. I was extremely relieved and he was profusely apologetic to both me and our leaders, who had now gathered round to see what the fuss was about.

He told us that the woman's son had been in the British army and was killed in an accident. Without asking, my spattered breakfast was replaced. So, during my little ordeal, nothing had escaped his eye. "Eat up lads, the show is over."

~

Many years later, the wonderful Father Ted TV comedy series dispersed any reservations I may have had about the Irish. Humour, and the ability to laugh at ourselves, is the greatest healer. In that series we were also repeatedly exposed to another word: feck. What a difference a letter makes. The "e" had blunted the great, "u"-laden, unutterable. But I'm sure that was not the intention behind my Irish harpy's surprising "o" version. I know that's what she said. It's seared in my memory. But then, memories can be fockle.

Chapter Four

St. Blaise and the Art of Veterinary Science

*We must welcome the future, remembering that soon it
will be the past; and we must respect the past,
remembering that it was once all that was humanly
possible.* – George Santayana

Modern veterinary science began with the founding of
the world's first veterinary school, the Royal Academy
of Lyons, by Louis XV, in 1761. It was a response to
the appalling livestock losses France suffered between
1710 and 1770 from epidemics of Cattle Plague (a virus
disease, also known as Rinderpest). Soon, another
school was established at the famous Maisons Alfort
near Paris. Other European countries followed France's
lead. The London Veterinary School dates from 1792.

How much I owe to *La Belle France*! Louis XV
was no less a persecutor of my Huguenot ancestors than
his royal predecessors; so it seems ironic that my
chosen career owes its origins to him—or perhaps to his
mistresses, Mme de Pompadour and Mme du Barry,
who are said to have held undue influence during the
latter part of his reign.

Unfortunately, these early veterinary schools had
neither the knowledge nor skills to influence the course
of epidemics like Cattle Plague. Until they began to
apply scientific principles, from the middle of the
nineteenth century, the principal treatments for animal
diseases tended towards dramatic interventions such as
bleeding, or cauterisations with hot irons that did more
harm than good. Bleeding was well documented even in
Roman times. It took two thousand years for more

rational procedures to displace what was little more than misplaced showmanship.

Edward Coleman, one of the founding professors of the London school, published a booklet: *Instructions for the use of Farriers attached to the British Cavalry and the Honourable Board of Ordinance.*

His treatment for "mad staggers" sets the tone:

The horse should lose at least four quarts of blood, and repeated every four hours during the first twelve, if the symptoms be not relieved. The top of the head should be blistered (the hair first being cut close), one ounce and a half of laxative powder... should be given immediately, or even two ounces if the horse be large. The hair should be cut off from the hoof to the fetlock joints, and boiling water poured on the part; this should be repeated twice in the day. Clysters [enemas] of warm water and salt should be given every two hours (one pound of salt to five quarts of water). If the horse does not purge in thirty-six hours after the first powder has been given, repeat the dose as before. Two rowels should be placed under his belly.

Rowels were pieces of leather forced through incisions to lie under the skin. The idea was to cause a severe infection and discharge of pus—draining away "evil humours".

In defence of early vets, Coleman was a human surgeon before he undertook to lead the fledgling British veterinary profession. He held his post at London for forty-five long years: far too long in the opinion of many. His advice for "mad staggers" in horses shows no advance over the treatment given more than one hundred years earlier to Charles II prior to his death in 1679. He was, literally, tortured to death by the well-intentioned ministrations of his royal physicians. It has been estimated that a total of fifty-eight drugs were given to him over his last five days. He was purged, bled, cauterised and clystered. Red hot irons were applied to his skull and feet. His urinary tract was inflamed by cantharides, an infusion of toxic metals in white wine was given as an emetic, and white hellebore sneezing powder was used to clear his nose. Modern physicians suspect that he suffered from a renal condition. Only a kidney transplant could have saved him.

Earlier still, during the Dark Ages, there was no pretence of rationality. Superstition reigned supreme. Anglo Saxon texts describe sorcery. To remedy illness caused by elves or demons one recipe recommended:

...a knife whose handle is made of the horn of an ox of tawny colour and which bears three bronze nails. Trace the mark of Christ on the forehead of the animals, as well as on each of its legs and then, in silence, pierce the left ear of the animal ...

However, some mediaeval treatments were simple, practical, and may have been successful. When Thomas, Archbishop of York was diagnosed with lovesickness in 1114, he was prescribed a bout of therapeutic lovemaking. Castration was also suggested—a rather more traumatic alternative. He spurned both options and died soon after.

Other prescribed cures were, of course, utterly imbecilic to our way of thinking and it would be a wonder if they were actually used, even four hundred years ago. Robert Burton (1577-1640), an Anglican clergyman, had a cure for depression that, were it proven effective today, would help to revive the flagging fortunes of the sheep industry. It involved boiling up the head of a virgin ram, removing and sprinkling the brains with herbs and then roasting them over hot coals. Three days exclusively on this diet, and the patient would be noticeably happier (or, for obvious reasons, claim to be). I'm sure that those responsible for marketing New Zealand lamb would not promote such an unlikely cure; but I do wonder if the efforts put into the marketing of deer velvet today—especially those proclaiming its aphrodisiac properties—are not built on equally spurious foundations.

Amongst seventeenth century superstitions was the belief in *sympathetic magic*. By this perverted logic the application of a salve to the object that caused an affliction would heal the affliction itself. Thus a salve, or ointment, applied to the weapon that caused an injury was regarded as more efficacious than treating the wound itself. Given some of the filthy preparations used to dress wounds in those days, this may well have been true.

Appealing to a saint presented a cheaper and far less daunting option than most of these primitive and painful remedies. Patron saints were asked to intercede, depending on their supposed powers. St. Apollonia had all her teeth pulled out with giant pincers when she was martyred, so she was a logical choice for those suffering from toothache; and those with diseases of the breast, quite naturally, sought St Agatha who had had her breasts cut off.

St. Blaise, Bishop of Sebaste in 4th century Armenia, was one of the most popular of the mediaeval saints. His image adorns church windows throughout Europe. He was the foremost veterinary saint. A ceremony is still held on St Blaise's Day, February 3rd, for the farmers of Naintré in France during which there is a mass and the gospel is read on behalf of their cattle.

St. Blaise is also the Patron Saint of throats because he once cured a boy who had swallowed a fish bone. A Benediction of the Throat is performed annually at St. Etheldreda's Church in London:

> *The minister requests those who desire their throats to be blessed to come forward to the altar rails. He then repeats St. Blaise's prayer, after which he takes two slender lighted candles, which have been blessed the previous day, Candlemas Day, and which are crossed and tied a few inches from the ends with a red ribbon so as to form a V, and places the V end of the candles beneath the chin of each suppliant, so as to touch both sides of the neck at once, saying at the same time: 'Per intercessionem S. Blasii liberet te Deus a malo gutturis et quovis alio male.'* (From *The Plague of the Phillistines.* See Bibliography.)

If you were suffering from diphtheria in the nineteenth century, before the advent of antibiotics, an appeal to a saint would certainly be safer than losing a pint of blood to a physician using his filthy fleam; although appealing to St. Blaise would seem to offer the risk of singed ears.

St. Blaise's intercessions were deemed to be especially potent for pigs and their diseases because he had once persuaded a wolf to return a pig—her sole possession—to a poor woman. Laugh all ye of little faith! But if you were a sick pig would you prefer someone praying for you, or to be on the receiving end of a jolly good rowelling courtesy of Professor Coleman?

Alas, despite all his miraculous cures, St. Blaise met a violent death. Agricolaus, the governor of Armenia, ordered him to be scourged, then to have his flesh torn by iron combs and, finally, to be beheaded. It sounds barbaric, but you don't have to scour today's papers too closely to come across similar injustices and atrocities.

~

You would expect, in these supposedly enlightened days, that people would seek a logical, scientific approach to the diagnosis and treatment of disease; but ignorance, superstition and brutality are always ready to surface, and the world is still awash with rampant charlatanism.

Mrs F, a client whose dog, a little Papillon called Alfie, suffered from fits, brought in a web page advertising a cure for epilepsy. It is widely accepted that even with modern drugs epilepsy can, at best, be managed: never cured. Alas, so it had proved for Alfie. His fits had increased in frequency and severity despite my best efforts. Laboratory tests had eliminated a host of possible underlying reasons for his distressing convulsions. Epileptic seizures stem from a malfunction in the electrical circuitry of the brain. This can be either as a result of brain injury and scarring, which may have occurred many years earlier, or as an inherited defect from parents. Even these congenital brain defects might not manifest themselves until the dog is several years old. Certain lines of certain dog breeds are known to be especially prone to inherited epilepsies.

In veterinary practice epilepsy is usually diagnosed by a process of ruling out other possible causes of "funny turns" such as imbalances of blood chemistry from kidney disease, lack of oxygen from heart valve defects, poisoning with lead or other toxins, or a viral or bacterial encephalitis. Once again, the clinical history is vitally important. In Alfie's case I needed to ascertain what he did before, during and after each fit; how long each fit lasted; how frequently they recurred; and whether any of his brothers or sisters suffered from fits.

A definitive diagnosis can be made from disrupted electrical brain wave patterns recorded on an electro-encephalogram (EEG). That would have been nice, but such equipment and the expertise to drive it are not to be found in small isolated towns like Otautau (where I spent much of my working life), or anywhere near them. On his history alone, I had a fair idea I was dealing with epilepsy.

Clinicians have always been reluctant to admit to ignorance. The less we know, the more we take refuge in jargon. Jargon of ancient provenance is particularly appealing. Why not fling in a bit of French—*petits mals* (little bads), *grands mals* (big bads)—before these charming classifications fall into disuse? Unfortunately, it was the big bads that were hitting Alfie.

Despite all we had tried by way of conventional therapy, Alfie was convulsing on a daily basis and for longer periods of time. His teeth clenched, his mouth foamed, his body arched in spasms, and his bowels voided. Each occasion left him weak and bewildered and his family, naturally, extremely distressed. Both Mrs F and I knew the time had come to put him out of his misery and let her and her family off the hook. Yet when Alfie came to the clinic for the last time, she clung to the downloaded printout. A "cure" for epilepsy was available on the Internet! You could order "Vet Select Seizure Formula" on line. The grammar and spelling tends to give these sites away. It claimed to be "veterinarian formulated" [I hate to see the noun, veterinarian, used as an adjective or adverb] and safe. The "all natural ingredients" included: "Bupleurum, peony, Tang-kuei, Scute, Chih-shih, Atractylodes, Licorice, Scorpion, Silkworm." Many more were listed: most as obscure and imaginary as the ones I've mentioned. Was the liquorice for flavouring and scorpion to give the mixture a bit of a sting in the tail? How many dog owners would be tempted to buy this mysterious formulation, lured by the aura of the unknown and the unknowable?

Was I arrogant to dismiss this remedy out of hand? I gently dissuaded Mrs F from trying it which, as an intelligent woman, she already knew in her own mind. Ultimately her heart followed and she was able to accept that, sadly, euthanasia was the best thing for Alfie and her family. Unsatisfactory as it was, it was the most humane course of action. How easy it is for the unscrupulous to give hope, where there is none, to those who desperately seek it.

I'm sure that many marketeers would hold this tidy little online business in high regard. Stuff the ethics, I hear them say … it uses the latest IT selling techniques and has great earning potential … "You can pay by Visa" and "we also accept online checks." A "Seizure Full Treatment Pack (240 capsules, 1oz. Seizure Homeopathic)" for only $83! Then that final cheery exhortation: "Add to basket!"

Unfortunately, those who do are contributing to the descent of our society into basket-case status. If quacks can make a living from such blatant exploitation of the desperate and gullible, it is a sad reflection on how poorly scientific thinking has penetrated modern society. It would be funny if it wasn't so downright frightening.

~

With Alfie I was dealing with a sensible and intelligent owner. However, there are times when, in the face of insuperable client-driven pressure, the modern vet must buckle and yield to the temptation of artifice or showmanship. Often this is when he is presented with a hopeless case. It was a lesson I learnt well from an older vet, Mike Harkness, when I did the rounds with him as a keen young student.

We had driven along the narrow twisting road towards Tebay to visit farmer DY's (Dour Yorkshireman's) sick cow. Every day for a week, we had brushed aside the sacking doorway and entered the gloom of the stone outbarn where she was housed. The musty, ancient air within was edged with the unmistakable taint of putrefaction. "Daisy" had severe pneumonia. Sulpha drugs, normally reliable, had failed. Daisy continued to run a temperature and lose weight. She wasn't eating in spite of mega injections of stinging intramuscular vitamins. "Parenterovite", a concentrated concoction of B vitamins, was an old favourite of Mike's. It came in glass phials and a knack was required to snap off the neck without lacerating your hands on the fine shards of glass. Mike, with unselfconscious showmanship, snapped the tops off cleanly and sucked the contents into a sterile glass syringe. Immediately, an intense aroma filled the air. I can only liken it to supercharged Marmite. The city slickers of that era—the late 1960s—doused themselves in Brut aftershave, but Parenterovite was Mike's trademark. It stained his hands and its sharp tang pervaded everything surrounding him. As we clambered into his Landrover each morning we became enveloped in a reeking womb of Parenterovite. It could have been worse. B vitamins are good masking agents for many of the evil smells in the veterinary world. Necrotic afterbirth, essence of footrot, stale dogs' pee on damp tweed: all yielded to the power of Parenterovite.

After four days Daisy was slowly failing. DY became doubly dour: DDY. Mike substituted the sulpha injections for a more expensive drug, penicillin. It was worth a try. DDY looked on pessimistically as with another "Whoa, l'al pet", Mike drove a large needle through her tough hide and discharged a syringeful of thick white magic into Daisy's wasting muscles. She gave only the merest groan of protest in her enfeebled state. Penicillin, the miracle drug, hadn't been around that long and people had high expectations about antibiotics; but they couldn't cure everything and Mike was well aware of this. A proud Yorkshireman himself, his accent broadened as he empathised with DY. The loss of a cow was serious on these small farms. Daisy represented 5 percent of DY's herd. He only had twenty milkers.

After a couple more days, Daisy's fever ebbed, but she continued to lose condition. When Mike peeled back the sacking rug, her ribs were prominent. He pulled out clumps of dull, matted hair and applied his stethoscope to her chest, encouraging me to listen too: "You'll not hear much worse than that, John". Daisy's lungs crackled and wheezed. But Mike also guided me to the areas over consolidated lung where there were no sounds at all. He explained about scarring "int'lungs", and painted a grave picture to DY of lungs honeycombed with pus. Even if she improved it was only likely to be a temporary remission. She would never be a productive animal again. He appealed to pragmatism. "Nay point in spending good money after bad. Hast'a considered t'knackers?" But DY wouldn't accept defeat. From greasy cloth cap to clarty clogs, he was an archetypical Dalesman. He clung grimly to a dying way of life on his remote smallholding. Stubbornness, resilience and determination were second nature to him. Mike understood, so he told DY about mustard poultices. In brief, a mustard paste was to be applied over Daisy's ribs and covered with brown paper, and held in place by the sacking cover. It wasn't such a far-fetched idea as it sounds: mustard plasters, or similar applications of heated antiphlogistene, a kaolin-based paste, applied to the chest, were commonly used by doctors on human patients—even into the 1920s. Who wouldn't grasp at any straw to treat pneumonia in the days before antibiotics? And if the patient didn't make it, at least they'd have died like Daisy: feeling warm int'chest.

Back in the Marmitesmobile, as we drove to our next call, Mike explained that the mustard poultice was unlikely to make any difference to Daisy's condition, but that it would give DY something to do, make him feel better, and allow him to come to terms with Daisy's inevitable demise. Bugger the science: such is the veterinary art. And we would move onto the next topic of conversation.

Mike, a deeply conservative man, was incensed about the impending introduction of decimalisation. His arguments against this were as emotive and irrational as his approach to his professional calling was not. "Twelve pennies in t' shilling is alreet ba me" he stormed. "It suits me to ha' a unit that's divisible by fower. Hast'a ever heard o' a cow wi' five tits?" But it was not really the maths that mattered to me. I was charmed by the language. "Hast'a?" in more formal Yorkshire parlance became "hast thou?" Thee, thou, thy. Why had these remnants survived in this corner of England?

The stone walls flashed by and at each turn of the lane, from our high seats in the Landrover, we glimpsed ancient stone farm buildings, flag-roofed and cobbleyarded, snuggled in the enfolding skirts of the high fells. I rejoiced that my prospective new career would shake me free from the grey uniformity of city life. Through Mike I was becoming aware that it would be about people as much as animals, feelings as much as facts, history as much as science. Though I had, at that stage of my life, never heard of St. Blaise, I now know that we would do well to remember him. Looking to the future is all very well, but we can enrich ourselves and more truly understand each other if we also have knowledge of our history.

The veterinary profession itself, which has faced many changes and grown stronger with each new challenge, has an interesting, if largely unheralded, history. Much of its past was intimately involved with one species: the horse.

Chapter Five

Equus Dissimile Est

Four things greater than all things are, -
Women and Horses and Power and War.
- Rudyard Kipling, "The Ballad of the King's Jest"

The early veterinary colleges in Europe were established because of concerns about the thousands of cattle dying from plagues. Considering the general level of ignorance about disease in the eighteenth century, initially there would have been very little that they could have contributed. Overwhelmingly, their experience would have been with horses, not cattle.

For centuries horses had occupied our lives to a degree we now find difficult to imagine. The numbers involved in public transport alone, were quite staggering. In 1904 The Royal College of Veterinary Surgeons met with representatives of the London General Omnibus Company and other local owners, to discuss how to control glanders. Between them they possessed around 145,000 horses. [Glanders is a nasty and usually fatal bacterial infection of horses, mules, donkeys and occasionally humans. It has now been eliminated from most western countries.]

At the end of the nineteenth century the first "horseless carriages" were appearing. As they progressively displaced horses, they significantly reduced the volume of horse work available for vets. The age of the horse, as a means of mass transport, was rapidly closing. By 1906 there were estimated to be about six hundred motor buses running in London: and as they increased exponentially, horse numbers plummeted.

In August 1911 *The Veterinary Record* (the journal of the British Veterinary Association) reported that the London General Omnibus Company was selling off horses at the rate of one hundred a week, and expected to have taken their remaining ninety-four horse-omnibuses off the road by the following month. A few months later, in the same journal, veterinarians themselves were extolling the virtues of motor cars as necessary adjuncts to veterinary practice.

Nevertheless, horses continued to play a major transport role throughout Britain, until the First World War. At the time my ancestors in Liverpool ran a modest bakery business, John Hicks Limited. Because they dealt with cereal grains, they also ran a side business as provender (animal feed) merchants. There were no pastures to loose your horses onto in a big city so, in a sense, the provender merchant was the petrol station of its day: providing the fuel that drove the horses.

The balance sheet for John Hicks Ltd. on the 5th November 1913 lists 51 horses, carts and harnesses as assets, at a total value of £573. Five horses were purchased for £149/10/- and seven were sold or disposed of for £150/10/-. One van was bought for £65. By 1924 the firm was fully motorised and the provender sales had become negligible. There would have been hundreds of similar-sized businesses throughout Liverpool and much of the western world, all converting to mechanical "horsepower" at around the same time.

Aside from their declining civilian role, horses had one last, tragic, fling serving on the battlefields of the First World War as cavalry mounts, as packhorses carrying machine guns, ammunition and supplies, or as draught horses pulling artillery, ambulances and supply wagons. It has been estimated there were 16 million horses involved on all fronts. Half of them died from injuries, disease, overwork, poisoning or exposure and, largely because of the risk of them bringing in "exotic disease", many of the remainder were shot or left behind rather than repatriated at the end of the war. This was a sad ending, especially when close bonds had developed between the horses and their handlers after years on campaign. In a rather poignant reminder of this Colonel Reakes, director of Veterinary Services and Remounts (New Zealand Veterinary Corps), wrote:

Before the home-coming embarkation from Egypt, there was many a sad parting between man and horse-mates in the hard years of war. The ill-usage of some horses that had been sold to callous Egyptians had convinced the New Zealanders that a merciful death was a better fate for a horse than bondage to a pitiless taskmaster, and numbers [of them] *for which kind owners were not available were given a painless death.*

The role of horses in war was almost at an end. Horses and horsemen were superseded by the tanks, armoured cars and warplanes which had wrought so much havoc amongst them in this brutal conflict.

For many of the craftsmen and trades people who relied on horses for a living, the early twentieth century would have been a period of profound change and hardship. Blacksmiths turned into motor mechanics; ostlers (stablemen) vanished so completely as to drop from the language; farriers, harness makers, hay and corn merchants, had to adjust: as did veterinarians. But vets were fortunate in that they could switch their focus onto other species. From this point on, it is possible to trace the rise and rise of small animal (pet) practice.

However, even if the horse as a working animal has largely disappeared, it will long remain for recreational purposes: in the racing industry, for show-jumping, eventing and endurance riding—and then there are the pony clubs. Consequently, horses still retain a place in the veterinary repertoire and a significant part of my veterinary training was dedicated to equine matters.

When I was a student, even in the late 1960s, horses, above all other domesticated animals, carried the mystique encapsulated by an older generation of Latin-literate vets in the catch-phrase *equus dissimile est*—the horse is different. Horses had been the cornerstone of the veterinary profession for so long that they were regarded differently from the other domesticated animals. Some students deemed it a far nobler thing to study the horse than impregnate their minds with trivia about inferior species. Once acquired, this form of snobbery, in my experience, is a life-long prejudice that persists post graduation. Some specialist horse vets know they carry a divine imprimatur denied to lesser vets who grub a living from farm work or, worse still, by tending dogs, cats and other small animals.

In any general veterinary text books available to my generation the section on horses occupied the position of first rank. My Sisson and Grossman *Anatomy of the Domestic Animals* (1964) devotes seventy eight pages dedicated to the skeleton of the horse, but only twenty-six to that of the "ox". The sheep is dismissed in a mere six pages; the pig in nineteen, and the dog in twenty-one. The cat does not exist. Feminists should draw no conclusions about the fifteen pages devoted to the magnificent genitalia of the stallion when only eight are allocated to those of the mare.

One of my favourite university textbooks was *Practical Animal Husbandry* by Miller and Robertson. This was first published in 1934 and I had the devil's own job securing the 1959 edition for my second-year studies. It contains wonderful diagrams with all sorts of block and tackle techniques for hobbling and restraining horses. One is entitled "Raising a Fallen Horse with Two Farm Carts"; in the background is the faint outline of an old-fashioned hayrick complete with thatched top. It quotes Sir Walter Scott, no less, on separating fighting dogs which are locked together *...they can only be separated by choking them with their own collars, till they lose wind and hold, or by surprising them out of their wrath by sousing them with cold water...* There are reams of sensible sexist advice about all aspects of animal handling, such as moving animals along a road: *If you are in charge of animals and have a man available, send him forward to warn traffic...*

Miller and Robertson also included a full section on washing the "yard" which is, in fact, the penis—in this case, of a horse. This is another euphemism of ancient provenance, well, at least three hundred years, because Samuel Pepys used it in his famous diary. In their description of washing the yard, Miller and Robertson also emphasised the importance of removing all the *smegma*. What a smackingly satisfying word to describe the offensive and irritating concretion of dried mucus and cells which build up beneath the horse's prepuce (foreskin)! A veterinary degree is a wonderful way to acquire arcane vocabulary and smegma is almost up there with *borborygmi* (the gurgling sounds made by the movement of fluid and gas through the intestines). In fact, I like them both so much that I shall take the opportunity to use them gratuitously in a later chapter.

Smegma, disappointingly, lacks the patina of long usage; being only of early nineteenth century origin but it is, indisputably (Oxford Dictionary), derived from the Greek word for soap. I suspect that the similar name shared by an excellent brand of kitchen whiteware is unconnected but, there again, with these continental brands, you never know. Smegma has a certain ring to it, but I can see why they chose a shortened version.

Before I entered university to commence my veterinary training, I had stayed on farms and spent many holidays with our local vet, Mr Betts, who worked in one of Liverpool's sooty suburbs. Aintree excepted, Liverpool is not recognisably a hub of the equine world and Mr Betts dealt almost entirely with dogs and cats. I'd had very little exposure to the horse world.

The Liverpool University Veterinary Faculty required its students to broaden their experience during the long summer vacations in the early pre-clinical years of the five year course by working on farms, in kennels, at abattoirs, stables or agricultural research facilities. To rectify my ignorance of all things equine I chose to spend my first university vacation at a riding establishment in a leafier part of my grimy home town. It wasn't a bad choice. One of my friends, Tony, spent the summer watching cattle being pole-axed and butchered on the floor of a primitive abattoir in Derby. Another, Richard, was consigned to painting colour coded dung cans at a research centre for some parasitological experiment. He learned that there is drudgery at the heart of even the greatest scientific endeavours. Meanwhile, I learned a lot about the complexities of human nature.

I don't think I ever worked out quite what was going on at the O'Reilly's, but they were certainly pleased to have my unpaid labour for a few weeks. The horses were kept in loose boxes and had to be "mucked out" daily. This was to be my job. Miller and Robertson gives precise instructions: ...*the clean portions* [of the straw removed] *should, if the weather is fine, be dried in the sun, aerated and then laid out in windrows across the direction of the prevailing winds; the windrows should be turned once or twice a day. On very wet or very windy days the clean bedding should be left in the passage behind the horses and the windows and doors kept open; if this is not possible... it is usual to remove only dung and soiled bedding, two or three times daily in a wicker basket emptied into a stable barrow outside.... Each layer of straw should be laid at right angles to the last...* Oh for the days before plastic displaced wicker and labour was cheap! To the O'Reillys of course, I was cheap labour. Even so, they had pared the ritual of windrows and aeration to a bare minimum. They were likeable rogues who slotted neatly into one of the stereotypes we all hold of the horse-savvy Irish. They weren't the sorts to do it by the book, but they knew their horses and they definitely weren't short of horse-dealer cunning.

When I first arrived, Tom, a precocious late teenager—roughly my own age, but infinitely more worldly—perfunctorily showed me the ropes. It was obvious that he was not particularly interested in doing this and that he had his mind on other things. He was openly "courting"—a less genteel word comes to mind—Sheila, the owner's daughter. There were convenient haylofts and thickets scattered round the property for such dalliances, as the need arose. In fact, the O'Reilly establishment would have made an ideal set for the filming of a DH Lawrence novel and, even if Tom had never heard of the great novelist, as he almost certainly hadn't, he was instinctively playing a lead role. He blithely ignored the advice attributed to a famous actress, Mrs Patrick Campbell: *I don't mind where people make love, so long as they don't do it in the street and frighten the horses.*

Some would have considered Sheila a coarse prize, and Tom appeared to treat her as such, but she was a willing hack for routine practice. I tried to look at it from his point of view. He was gaining experience from an older mare, perhaps past her best, but leaving his options open should a superior mount become available. He certainly kept a look-out for any promising young fillies that came his way.

One such was the divinely svelte Perdita. Her name alas, when massacred by the Liverpool accent, lost its classical pretensions—the last syllable becoming a choked sneeze: Paair/dee/cha. Perdita was one of those horse-mad young girls who festoon riding stables the length of Britain. I was not immune to her lissom figure, for I was a late maturing adolescent: an innocent soul awash in my sea of hormones. In my testosterone-twisted fantasies Perdita readily qualified as a Greek goddess, albeit one with a Latin name.

Women, so we are told, admire confidence in a man above all other traits; and Tom—in spite of, or, perversely, because of, his other rather obvious conquest—had Perdita in his thrall. There was no doubt in my mind that he was grooming her for future adventures.

How could I not envy Tom his carefree nature and animal magnetism? He reaped New Testament rewards for Old Testament sins, for had not Jesus said: *...unto everyone that hath shall be given; and from him that hath not, even that he hath shall be taken away...*? And thus, in biblical terms, ingrained from a thousand attendances at school chapel, I contrasted his love life with mine.

If I were to be perfectly honest, and cast all adolescent envy aside, I had to admit that Tom had the makings of a superb horseman. I was to witness this one day when a mare—securely tied to an iron ring in a wall—was spooked by the sirens of passing fire engines. Tensed and unable to break free she became a vision of captive terror, several hundred kilos of hide-bound grenade: muscle, bone and sinew. Her hooves sparked as they struck the drive: a toe-crushing tap-dance of iron on concrete. She arched backwards, straining as she wove from side to side on the taut rope: a fish fighting on thin line.

Something would have parted—a violent avulsion, with risk of injury to horse and bystanders—had not Tom appeared. With no hesitation or hint of concern for his personal safety, he laid his arms round the bunched muscles of her neck and, embracing her with calming words, drew himself towards her as to a lover in tormented anguish; and oh so gently!

The great creature relaxed. The moment passed. Her head dropped in soothed submission, and all was well. It was an exhibition of naked courage. Tom had simultaneously demonstrated the depths of his genuine and instinctive love for his horses and semaphored his capabilities as a different sort of lover to any admiring females who happened to have seen his heroic display.

Mucking out each morning at the O'Reilly's was a breeze, save for Bruno, the gelding in one loose box. I was warned to be especially careful about him. He

56

could well be a rig, in fact they almost certainly knew he was. (A rig is a horse with a retained testicle and which, consequently, looks like a gelding but behaves like a stallion). The funny thing was, once Bruno was saddled up, he behaved perfectly.

The O'Reillys, as I later discovered, were trying to sell Bruno before he killed someone. The moment you approached his stable door he laid his ears back and swung his powerful hindquarters towards the door as if to say "Get past me if you can, mate!" Tom had instructed me to be briskly efficient in such situations. I must always show the horse who was boss. Since I had been entrusted with the task I wasn't going to grovel back to Tom each time I ran into difficulties. Besides, *I* had the Greek goddess to impress, and *he* had the habit of disappearing for long stretches of time. Which thicket was I to look behind?

I managed to complete the mucking out successfully, if with some trepidation, for several days. But one morning Bruno seemed to be in a more menacing mood than usual. His rear end swayed warningly as I reached for the bolt to undo his stable door. His ears were flat down on his neck. I talked to him—as advised by Miller and Robertson: *when approaching a horse, whether in a stall or a loose box, always speak to it before touching it*. More to reassure myself than Bruno, I said, "You might be in a swinish mood today, old chap, but I'm going to clean out your box—come what may", or words to that effect. Bruno had other ideas. *Approach from the left side and handle the head or neck first*. I agreed with Miller and Robertson, I needed to try and get to his neck, put a head collar on him and lead him outside. But it was easier said than done, the only access was from the rear and it was well guarded by his hefty hindquarters.

There was no advice about getting to the head and neck under such circumstances. Perhaps you should employ "a man" to do it for you. *It is better to treat a strange horse with suspicion, but do not let it suspect that you are afraid of it.* Yes, yes, yes! So now was the time to show it who was boss? Confidently I raised my broom, commanded him to move over in my sternest voice, and thwacked the brush end against his massive gluteals. It was a big mistake yet, at the same time, an immensely instructive moment. Instantaneously, two panels of the solid tongue-and-grooved door between us were shattered at the height of my groin. I had not even had time to withdraw my broom. It clattered ineffectually on the floor beneath the stamping steel of his hooves. At this stage I decided to ignore Miller and Robertson and left Bruno to stew in his own juice. One of the O'Reillys would have to deal with him later.

Mrs J had ridden Bruno several times and he seemed to be all she desired of a horse. Unwisely, she had never visited him to catch and saddle him up herself. Whenever she rang to make an appointment to ride Bruno, the kind people at O'Reilly's always had him ready for her. She was considering buying him and was visiting for one last ride that afternoon. Mr O'Reilly instructed Tom: "She's coming at two. Get the bastard saddled up by half-one. With luck she'll make up her mind this time." I would have felt worse about my failure that morning if it hadn't taken three of us to distract and coax Bruno from the loose box where I had left him but, deep down, I knew that Tom would have managed by himself.

In due course the deal was made. Mrs J was upset that the O'Reillys were unable to provide livery for her new acquisition, but she had made alternative arrangements and rode off happily enough. Everybody at O'Reillys' breathed more easily. Bruno was off their backs at last.

I felt sorry for Mrs J, she seemed a decent sort, but there is no room for naivety when you're buying a horse. Nothing more was heard from her, but as to whether that was because she was satisfied with her deal, reluctant to complain, or had already appeared among the death notices of *The Liverpool Echo*—I felt it imprudent to enquire.

Perdita, my little goddess, remained unimpressed and indifferent towards me, but that was all right. In this spring of my youth it was great to be alive. The world was full of beautiful, summery women and every day I saw a goddess or two. I could never be a Tom, nor did I want to be. I acknowledged, however misguidedly, that I was a romantic, and I didn't care for coarse rumpy and, deep down, I knew that one day I would find a goddess who was interested in me. And very soon, I did.

Chapter Six

King Alfred and the Pied Piper of Watling Street

Grave old plodders, gay young friskers,
Fathers, mothers, uncles, cousins,
Cocking tails and pricking whiskers,
Families by tens and dozens,
Brothers, sisters, husbands, wives --
Followed the Piper for their lives.
– Robert Browning: The Pied Piper of Hamelin.

In the event, the goddess I found had equine connections in the form of a much-loved pony whose full name was Coffee Cariad (the last name being Welsh for darling). He and I competed on unequal terms for her attentions. While he was petted and pampered in a field near the Lanfear's house in Radlett, just north of London, I was suffering the rigours of my demanding university course nearly two hundred miles away in Liverpool. While Coffee yielded to the delights of long grooming sessions with dandy brush, curry comb and hoof pick, I was sequestered in a small student bedsit poring over dense texts or cramming for tests and exams—pining for my next encounter with Coffee's winsome owner and those sweet moments when the drudgery of existence would be effaced by her loving companionship.

Whenever possible I made the trip south and, I have to concede, Viv occasionally forsook Coffee and travelled to Liverpool. For the first year of our courtship we made these journeys by rail but, on my twenty-first birthday, I was given a green Morris Minor by my parents. I felt immensely privileged, and slightly guilty because of it, but I was now free to beetle down to Radlett whenever I could.

The start and finish of the drive weren't too demanding. I picked up the M6 outside Liverpool, came off it somewhere near Stafford to catch the A5, and trundled across the Midlands to join the M1 near Coventry. In those days there was no motorway link between the M6 and M1.

The A5 is an ancient highway, still known by its Saxon name of Watling Street. In the ninth century it marked part of the boundary to which Alfred the Great, from his stronghold in Wessex, had rolled back the invading Vikings. South and west of Watling Street was Alfred's Anglo-Saxon kingdom; north and east of it was the area administered by the Danes. On modern maps Watling Street drives, as straight as when it was built by the Romans, through what is now a densely populated area of England. Where the legions once marched in orderly files behind their proud standards now, nearly two thousand years later, lorries thundered along a three-lane highway spewing their acrid blue fumes. During the early 1970s the A5 was, until the M45 link was finally completed, a dangerous bottleneck on the major route connecting north with south, and it was regularly disrupted by delays for road works and traffic accidents.

One sombre winter's afternoon, as the beetle and I reluctantly headed back to Liverpool, we stumbled on the police just as they were starting to close off the A5 near Cannock. I cursed my luck, for we were the first to be diverted. There was a detour sign and I followed the arrow, assuming that we would soon be directed back onto the A5. But, perhaps typically, after a couple of signs the trail petered out. Assuming I must have missed one, I pulled over to the side of the rather minor road where I now found myself, and studied my trusty AA road atlas. It was disconcerting to know that I had not the foggiest idea where I was. I felt a bit like the unfortunate tourist lost in Ireland who asked a local the way to Tipperary. "Now if I was going to Tipperary" the local is purported to have answered, "I wouldn't have started from here!" Where the f*** were we? A large truck pulled up behind me. He was blocking the road, but seemed strangely content to sit there.

From early childhood I had been encouraged to map read and, in the fading light, I hazarded a guess about our location and plotted a likely escape route for my little beetle and me down some narrow-looking country lanes. Road atlases have their deficiencies, one of them being that they don't show every minor road. The large truck started up as soon as I took off. We hadn't travelled very far before I was following my nose. Perhaps the truck driver was lost, too? I became more convinced as he stuck on my tail down one improbable turn after another. Unless by some remarkable coincidence Truckie also had plans to go to the middle of the same nowhere as me, on this gloomy Sunday evening, I was not alone in my predicament. I became increasingly aware that I was leading him astray. Surely he would be starting to feel a bit suspicious, perhaps even a tad annoyed? I decided to press on with confidence rather than risk stopping again.

The narrow lane I finally chanced on was a distinct gamble. It looked suspiciously like a farm track and soon, just as I feared, it ended in a farmyard. It wasn't easy with Truckie on my tail, but I managed a quick three point turn and shot back past him in the direction we'd just come. Straight away, I was confronted by what his looming presence and the deep-hedged lanes had been concealing—an army of followers. Even with my little Morris Minor it was a tight squeeze getting past the long queue on that narrow farm track for, scattered among the family saloons, was a fairly representative sample of the heavy vehicles which keep the wheels of industry turning: a concrete mixer, two car transporters, assorted removal vans and some earth-moving equipment. I didn't stop. It was starting to get dark and besides, imagine what would have happened to me when they found out that I wasn't the farmer departing his farm for a jolly evening out at the local pub, but the idiot who had led them there! With luck, that accolade would fall on the driver of the truck who had so foolishly assumed that I knew where I was going.

When I got back to Liverpool later that night and watched the late night news, I was not in the least surprised to learn that there was a major traffic jam in the Midlands which, it was anticipated, would take the authorities several more hours to clear. I wondered why they weren't talking days. I still wonder how they managed to extract those behemoths of industry, many of them articulated and difficult to reverse, from such a tight spot, so quickly.

~

For two more years our courtship played out across those congested miles. At the end of my third year we were married and living in happy penury. Two more years of hard work lay ahead of me before I could earn my first salary as a qualified vet—always assuming I passed all my exams. During my final year I was a kept man while Viv held down a job she detested, behind the counter of a Building Society.

Watling Street had been a lifeline, so I have a certain fondness for it and an admiration for the Romans who built it. I wonder what Alfred, that inspired Saxon king, would have thought of the choking, polluted highway that once formed the boundary of his nation. Where were the pure streams and the deep forests full of game? What spreading cancer of bricks, concrete and asphalt now laid waste his realm? Would he be able to endorse Shakespeare: *this scepter'd isle… This precious stone set in the silver sea…?*

I had my doubts and, in due course, they played a part in our decision to emigrate to New Zealand. We never guessed that New Zealand would be where we were to spend the greater part of our working lives and bring up our family. But, much as we love New Zealand, the scepter'd isle is buried in our psyches. Our roots go too deep. I can't shake off that past and neither can Viv. We have given up trying, for in coming to New Zealand we have become doubly enriched, and now lay claim two spiritual homes: the ancient land of our birth and the beautiful land of our adoption.

Chapter Seven

Krebs and Quills

Thousands of years ago, cats were worshipped as gods. They have never forgotten this. – Anon

Despite my boyhood indiscretions, in my professional life I have ministered to cats with all due care and attention. I overcame my ingrained prejudices and for a few years Viv and I owned a cat—in so far as anyone can ever lay claim to owning one. Moon was a much-loved pet, but definitely of the common, moggy variety. But my *volte-face* only went so far. I could never describe myself a cat fancier. Before a chocolate point Siamese or apricot Persian ever reached my examination room table, I made every effort to know precisely which breed was being presented to me and how his or her colour was to be described: silver or blue, never grey; red—so much more exotic than brown. My receptionists were trained to ask these questions and write them on the pet's card so that I did not suffer the ignominy of failing to recognise a detail that was likely to be of utmost importance to the owner.

I was so much ahead of my colleague Daryl in this regard. His house was crawling with cats. He loved them. Yet he could never be bothered with these details. All cat fanciers are cat lovers, but Daryl is proof that the reverse doesn't necessarily hold true. He wouldn't have recognised a Rex from a Ragdoll and filled in the "breed" section of the patient card with one word: "Alley". Understandably, this did not endear him to genuine Cat Fancy people even though he never dealt with their exotic "alley cats" with anything less than due care. As for me, I must redeem the catapulting sins of my childhood with the tale of Max, a Persian—a "proper" cat.

Some people would, quite correctly, dismiss Persians as long-haired genetic freaks to whom cat fanciers have given an exotic and misleading appellation. They have imposed breed standards that specify the deformity of brachycephaly (squashed-in faces) to give an appealing wide-eyed, round-faced look. As a direct result Persians are predisposed to tooth problems, corneal injuries and infections, and facial eczemas. Their dim wittedness, gentle natures and a propensity to other medical problems (of which bladder stones are but one example), make them a vets' delight.

They are the very opposite of the typical cogger's moggy. Max, like most other Persian cats, would have been totally incapable of supporting himself in the wild, under which designation I include the sooty wilds of Liverpool. His long, matted coat would have snagged on the broken bottles that many people cemented onto the top of the brick walls—a common strategy in Liverpool to deter vandals and burglars—whereas "pure bred" alley cats floated over them with ease.

During the long course of Max's treatment Viv and I became great friends with his owners and, I must concede, Max was a bit of a character. When we left to go overseas we were extremely fortunate that Moon, our low born alley cat, was eagerly adopted into their cat-loving family and accepted by her new brother without prejudice, even though he must have known that she wasn't a "proper" cat.

Max suffered from a complaint that has afflicted man and beast for centuries: bladder stones.

An eternal cycle of complex chemical interactions rages within the tissues of our bodies. As a student I was always aghast to see the wall-poster mapping out all the biochemical reactions known to be involved in "Krebs' cycle", the process by which we derive energy from food. It was as colourful as a London Underground map but infinitely more complicated. Arrows marked the transformation of one multi-syllabic molecule into another. Enzymes italicised this busy scene, with curved arrow interferences. I have always had a morbid fear of flow charts, so I preferred to regard it as a work of art rather than something I would need to understand in detail. Indeed it was, and still is, a work in progress. If that 1970s map would have occupied the top of a decently sized kitchen table, the modern version, plumped up with the biochemical advances of the last forty-five years, has expanded to occupy an the area the size of a barn door.

Something, somewhere on Max's map had gone wrong and Max could no longer urinate freely. Stones were blocking his urinary tract: perhaps triggered by an infection which had altered the acidity of his urine, or a mineral imbalance in his diet of cat biscuits, or even a reluctance to drink enough to keep his urine diluted sufficiently. The pathology of urinary stone formation is complex; but the crystals precipitating out in Max's bladder had formed a gritty, sandy obstruction in his urethra—the fine and delicate tube draining the bladder to the outside.

The problem for any male cat suffering from this quite common condition, is that grit accumulates near the tip of the penis which, in cats, is the narrowest part of the urethra. Max went around straining to pass urine, but his only reward was a few blood-tinged drips on his owners' favourite candlewick bedspread. It really is a very fiddly job to grasp a cat's penis, let alone insert a fine catheter into the minute orifice and flush the sand away. Even if the vet manages to restore the full bore candlewick spraying service, and makes changes to his patient's diet and lifestyle to try and modify the faulty Krebs' factors, the condition tends to recur.

There is a surgical treatment: perineal urethrostomy. The name, admittedly, is a mouthful, but sometimes it is advisable to disguise acts of surgical barbarism with euphemistic Latinisms. What owner is going to appreciate your recommendation to "chop the penis off" a beloved pet? Whichever way it is described, amputation of the tip of the penis removes the bottleneck. After consultation with Max's owners, this delicate operation was duly performed. The wider bore urethra behind the penis was anchored with fine silk stitches to his perineal skin, leaving a larger opening through which those gritty stones could pass. Max was already castrated, so it is doubtful that he missed what had become a superfluous and bothersome piece of his anatomy.

Max was fine for a while, but he did have some trouble with skin at the site of the operation overgrowing his new orifice—a process known as epithelialisation. This can be managed with periodic re-catheterisation and stretching. In Max's case my timing was immaculate because we left the district soon after his operation, and while Max was in full working order. As the successful surgeon it fell on me to savour the adulation of his doting owners. Some other poor unfortunate vet was left with his tricky aftercare and the fiddly re-catheterisations periodically required to keep him in full flow.

~

The seraglios of the Levant provide an interesting historical aside to this very problem. It is common knowledge that through the ages the harems of Eastern gentlemen were guarded by eunuchs. In most cases these were castrated men. However, there was also a class of eunuchs who suffered the supreme indignity of having their penises amputated. In this case, it seems, they were, literally, "chopped off". The losses to such primitive surgery from blood loss and infection were staggering, but those who survived had the same problem with stricture as Max. Without polyethylene catheters how did they manage? The answer, apparently, was goose quills—far more acceptable to those who prefer biodegradable alternatives. Armed with this knowledge you would now know, were you to enter a time warp and come across a mediaeval Arab with a goose quill tucked in his turban, not to make the mistake of assuming he was a scribe.

So much for the distal urethra: anatomists love to sprinkle their descriptions of body parts with Latin or Greek locators: rostral, caudal, palmar, plantar, lateral, medial, distal, proximal. The distal urethra is the part furthest from the body. The next part of our journey plunges proximally along this delicate and sensitive organ, to an area rich in historical associations.

Chapter Eight

Intolerable Urethral Intrusions

March 26th 1667 *"...I have cause to be joyful this day, as being my usual feast-day for my being cut of the stone this day nine years; and through God's blessing am at this day and have long been in as good condition of health as ever I was in my life..."* The Diary of Samuel Pepys

There is little time during the busy five-year veterinary curriculum to reflect on the history of medicine. Many years passed before I realised that my little foray into urinary tract surgery was not without historical precedents, but Thomas Hollier's name will live longer than mine, even though his surgery was performed more than 300 years earlier. His patient, the famous Samuel Pepys, has ensured that.

The unbalanced diets and lifestyles of the seventeenth century English frequently led to gout and "stone". However, like Max, Samuel Pepys' stone probably involved an inherited defect in one of his biochemical pathways. We can deduce this because both Pepys' mother and aunt suffered from "stone". This inherited predilection would have been exacerbated by his less than restrained lifestyle.

On March 26th 1658 Pepys, a young man of twenty-five who had yet to begin his famous diary, underwent surgery to remove the stone from his bladder. Apparently there were several barber surgeons offering this service, so it was a reasonably common procedure. Some patients lived, some died. Pepys was lucky. Thomas Hollier, his father's neighbour, was a skilled surgeon attached to St Thomas's Hospital. His record was better than most. He did thirty similar operations in the year he operated on Pepys, with no subsequent loss of life; yet in another year his first four patients died—almost certainly from post-operative infections. In the days before there was any appreciation of the need for surgical cleanliness, still less sterility, this was the greatest risk. There was no concept of asepsis, and neither patient nor surgeon were too concerned if the instruments were dirty and the surgeon's apron was, as has been recorded, stiff with dried pus. However, by having the operation performed in a private house, Pepys was probably spared some of the risk.

The prospect of being knifed and probed in such a delicate area without the benefit of an anaesthetic (still two hundred years from discovery), would have been quite terrifying. But Pepys had no choice: the pain and spasms associated with being unable to urinate properly are unendurable.

For analgesia Pepys was prescribed a soothing draught of liquorice, marsh mallow, cinnamon milk, rose water and white of eggs. And that, apart from mopping his brow as the scalpel sliced, is as far as it went.

The technique involved inserting a silver probe, or *itinerarium* (an unusual traveller), through the penis, along the urethra and into the bladder. The stone would be located when the probe was felt to grate against it. The surgeon could now make his incision, midway between the scrotum and anus, and cut down onto the tip of the probe in the neck of the bladder. A reasonably lengthy incision was required. Samuel Pepys' stone, by his description, was the size of a "tennis ball". Even allowing for the fact that it was "real tennis" that was played in those days, for which the ball was marginally smaller than that used in the modern game, an incision about three inches long would have been required. The stone was grasped with forceps and removed in less than a minute. The wound was not stitched, but left to drain and heal itself.

A similar method is used for the extraction of smaller stones in dogs, to this day; and some veterinary surgeons still recommend leaving the wound unstitched and left open to drain. That is the way I was taught, and as a demonstration of the healing powers of that portion of anatomy, a veterinary surgeon's faith in leaving it so is usually well rewarded. However, in Pepys's case it is thought that the wound never entirely healed and that his infertility could have been a consequence of this; not, as he well recorded, that it had any effect on his potency.

Here any parallels between Pepys and Max must be dispelled, for Max, being castrated, was a perfect gentleman. Pepys, on the other hand, behaved like a tom cat. Indeed, it is the disarming honesty with which he reveals his human frailties, and his associated guilt in indulging them, that make his diaries such a delight to read.

So Pepys was lucky, his operation was a success. He celebrated the anniversary of his operation each year and made frequent, grateful references in his diaries to his deliverance from his agonising complaint. He duly had his stone mounted in a case and, because he was meticulous about monetary affairs, we know that this cost him twenty-four shillings.

Pepys' curiosity knew no bounds and he had many influential contacts. In 1662 he records visiting the Hall of the Barber-Surgeons' Company and attending the dissection of a seaman who had been hanged for robbery:

I did touch the dead body with my bare hand; it felt cold, but methought it was a very unpleasant sight. But all the Doctors at table conclude that there is no pain at all in hanging, for that it doth stop the circulacion of the blood and so stops all sense and motion in an instant. Thence we went into a private room, where I perceive they prepare the bodies, and there was the Kidnys, Ureters, yard, [Remember? Pepys was not talking about his garden.] *stones and semenery vessels upon which he read today. And Dr. Scarborough upon my desire and the company's did show very clearly the manner of the disease of the stone and the cutting and all other Questions that I could think of.*

In 1628 Dr William Harvey had demonstrated the way blood circulated and the heart's action as a pump; but the role of nerves and the spinal cord in the transmission of pain to our conscious brain were unknown until an Anglican clergyman, Stephen Hales, started poking them around in decapitated frogs— sometime in the next century—experiments which even then provoked anti-vivisection protests. Pepys's learned friends' conclusions about the pain of hanging were, if correct, correct for the wrong reasons: a common failing of medical experts throughout the history of medicine.

~

While we are ensconced in the nether regions it would be remiss not to mention an operation of an even more horrific nature practised in Fiji and Tonga, as recorded in the first volume of that well known British medical journal *The Lancet*, (17th January 1834). In an article entitled *Traumatic Tetanus*, one R. Liston (presumably Robert Liston, the famous surgeon) uncritically transplanted a section from Mariner's book: *Voyage to the Tonga Islands.*

Tetanus, it appears was a very common disease among the natives of Fiji:

...who from their warlike habits, are more frequently in the way of it; they adopt, however, a remedy which the Tonga people have borrowed from them, and consists of the operation of tocolosi, *or passing a reed first wetted with saliva into the urethra, so as to occasion a considerable irritation and discharge of blood; and if the general spasm be very violent, they make a seton of this passage, by way of passing down a double thread looped over the end of the reed; and when it is felt in the perineum* [echoes of Hollier's itinerarium here] *they cut down upon it, seize hold of the thread, and withdraw the reed, so that the two ends of the thread hang from the orifice of the urethra, and the doubled part from the artificial opening in the perineum; the thread is occasionally drawn backwards and forwards, which excites very great pain and abundant discharge of blood.*

Liston claimed that thirty to forty per cent of cases of tetanus recovered as a result of tocolosi, but he was merely recycling Mariner's hearsay evidence. As a cure for tetanus, tocolosi makes no sense. It is medical rubbish.

While it is entirely possible that the pain produced by this barbaric procedure would be enough to evince signs of life from a near corpse, it is to be hoped that early nineteenth century English physicians were not, as a consequence of this gem in *The Lancet*, inspired to inflict tocolosi on any of their patients. However, the early nineteenth century was an age of untrammelled experimentation and large egos and it is entirely possible that they did.

Robert Liston (1794 – 1847), surgeon and anatomist, was described (by medical author Roy Porter) as ...*a lion of a man with a sharp knife and a sharper temper. Speed was his forte, biting his blade between his teeth like a butcher so as to free his hands to save time. Lithotomy* [stone removal]*, he declared, 'should not occupy more than two or three minutes at most'.*

It is possible to imagine this tall, powerful and celebrated man marching round to the editors of *The Lancet*, scalpel clenched between his teeth, demanding publication in their journal. How could they refuse?

Before anaesthetics, speed was of the essence. Liston's students were in the habit of timing his operations with their stopwatches. Whereas his fellow surgeons, in these days before anaesthetics, might require six men to restrain and assist with the amputation of a leg, Liston was strong enough to use only one. Operating with great speed and skill, he compressed the femoral artery with his left hand while doing all the cutting and sawing with his right.

It is sobering to realise that, almost until Liston's day, surgery had scarcely advanced over nearly two thousand years. Celsus, a Roman surgeon of the first century, described techniques of plastic surgery and, indeed, bladder surgery—including precise directions for crushing and removing stones. Celsus claimed that a surgeon should be ...*youthful or in early middle age, with a strong and steady hand, as expert with the left hand as the right, with vision sharp and clear, and spirit undaunted; so far void of pity that while he wishes only to cure his patient, yet is not moved by his*

cries to go too fast, or cut less than is necessary.
Someone, in fact, very like Liston.

From the mid nineteenth century, surgery and medical knowledge expanded rapidly. In December 1846 Liston, himself, performed the first major operation in Europe with the benefit of anaesthesia—a thigh amputation. At its successful completion he is supposed to have remarked, "Gentlemen, this Yankee dodge beats mesmerism hollow". However, the need for hygiene to prevent post-operative infections was still unrecognised. The death rate following limb amputations varied between 25 and 60 per cent in the 1850s and, in military practice, was as high as 90 per cent. Change in the army always came slowly. Dr John Hall, the Chief of Medical Staff of the British Expeditionary Army during the Crimean War, was an unpleasant character: a flogging disciplinarian who treated the troops like scum. He was vindictive and obstructive towards Florence Nightingale when she was lobbying for re-organisation of the inefficiently run and appallingly unsanitary military hospitals. In a letter of instructions to his officers at the start of the campaign he warned them against the use of chloroform. *The smart use of the knife is a powerful stimulant and it is much better to hear a man bawl lustily than to see him sink silently into the grave.*

There is a gruesome satisfaction to be had from reading these accounts and counting our blessings in the (perhaps false) belief that we live in a more enlightened age; or even to contemplate that while refined nineteenth century society languished in the regency drawing rooms of Bath, something far more vigorous was going on in coir huts on the other side of the world. What would the genteel Jane Austen have made of tocolosi? But medical knowledge would have remained static without these early and only partially controlled experiments on the human body.

Jane Austen had her own health problems. Medical historians have deduced that she died of Addison's disease. She was only forty-two. The study of endocrinology dates from 1849 when Dr Thomas Addison first described the condition named after him and showed that it was caused by disease of the adrenal glands.

Since my surgical interventions on Max's behalf, I have had a rather large taste of modern medicine and surgery myself, and it has given me the incentive to reflect on these things. With the wisdom of age I suggest that patient care would be immeasurably improved were surgeons put on the receiving end of their treatments before they were licensed to inflict them on others. Of course, this is an impractical notion: Robert Liston would have become hopping mad and, with repeated incursions, completely stumped.

When Viv and I returned to New Zealand from a stint in small animal (dog and cat) practice in Yorkshire, I was thirty. It had been a valuable eighteen months' experience for me, but our years in Taranaki and Ashburton had given us a taste for the more relaxed New Zealand lifestyle and, apart from the ordeal of re-separating from our families, we couldn't wait to return.

Chapter Nine

Southland and New Beginnings

Immigration is the sincerest form of flattery. – Jack Paar

When Viv and I returned from England there were only two vacancies for vets in the whole South Island, the place we dearly wanted to be. We could try either Hokitika on the West Coast, or for a locum position for six weeks in Otautau, Southland. It had to be Otautau because, as Viv said, "You know how I react to sandfly bites." The West Coast, although an area of outstanding interest and beauty, is well known for the voracity of its sandflies.

Like most New Zealanders, we knew little about Southland. I had imbibed the "frozen wasteland" propaganda reinforced in the minds of other Kiwis by the evening weather forecasts, and the negativity of Auckland-based travel agents. But Southland has areas of outstanding natural beauty and a fascinating past; and when you start to grasp the history of a place you begin to belong to it and feel at home.

Two years before Jane Austen's birth, Captain James Cook made his first landfall in the far south of New Zealand—among the fiords on its western edge. Fiordland was then—and still is—by far the wildest part of the country. The *Resolution* had spent four months probing deep into Antarctic waters in search of the great southern continent without success, and Cook decided to rest his crew ...*it must be natural for me to wish to injoy some short repose in a harbour where I can procure some refreshments for my people of which they begin to stand in need of....* So, on 26th March 1773, the great man brought his ship to anchor in the safe harbour of Dusky Sound—a place he had noted, but been unable to visit, on his earlier voyage (1768-1771) in the *Endeavour*. For five weeks he and his crew recovered and explored the area. The stumps of the trees he felled to clear an area for his astronomer's observatory are still identifiable at Astronomer Point. Many of the other place names he bestowed on local landmarks live on, and have replaced those by which they would have been known to the few Maori families he came across—such as the place of his first recorded encounter with them: Indian Island.

Dusky Sound retains the impress of history. Just over two-hundred years after Cook's visit, and after three days of rough tramping, I was thankful to lower the pack from my back, sit on the rocks outside the remote hut at Supper Cove and drink in the peace. It is a changeless place. Dark, dense forests cloak its steep shores. Bellbirds cast their clear tones across its glassy waters, much as Cook's crew would have heard them. The ghosts of his visit remain.

A keen imagination can people this emptiness, and the mere matter of two hundred years dissolves away in the eerie stillness of its cool mists ... rowlocks creak as men row ashore; light waves slapping the hollow planks; timber spars groan under damp ropes; a pungent waft of tar drifts from the men caulking the sprung timbers of their ship—wounded by the constant battering of the Great Southern Ocean. A fishing party sets out to explore. Their hoarse voices, hardened by months under sail, slur, become whispers and the scene fades …

I, too, shall have freshly caught fish for supper.

~

Otautau is a small town within a few kilometres, as the crow flies, of Captain Cook's lonely anchorage. However, in that short distance over the Fiordland mountains the landscape changes dramatically. If Cook had travelled east from Supper Cove, and crossed the rugged, bush-clad ranges, he would have reached a large and fertile plain of red tussock and tall forests.

Within a few decades of Captain Cook's early visits sealers and whalers were established on the south coast, intermarrying with local Maori. Before long they were tracking inland across the red-tussocked plains and following the inland hunting routes of the first inhabitants, the *tangata whenua*. From the seedling settlement of Riverton, they would have followed the Aparima River inland through Otautau, *the place of the greenstone pendant with the curved tip*. There was a thriving community here even in 1850, when the area was officially explored by a party from HMS Acheron.

The hunger for land in this new colony was explosive. By March 1857, John Turnbull-Thompson, the first Surveyor-General of New Zealand had completed his survey of the interior. During three short months he had, according to his great grandson and biographer, John Hall-Jones, *travelled over, mostly on foot, 1,500 miles of difficult country and had surveyed by reconnaissance two and a half million acres.* The total population of this vast area was 442, comprising 119 Maori and 253 Europeans and half-castes; before long it was claimed for agriculture. Over the next century the Southland plains were vigorously cleared and drained, creating a large area of what is now highly productive farmland.

~

In 1979 Viv and I drove from Invercargill late in the afternoon of a soft, spring day with some trepidation. What did Southland hold for us? To our relief the flat plains soon yielded to more rolling country. The Longwood hills now filled our horizon, their bush clad slopes light and dark: shadowed beneath fluffy cumuli, pierced by the shafts of a westering sun. Our road skirted around them and towards the distant dog-toothed Takitimus, a long, jagged range, representing the upturned canoe of Maori legend. The snows of winter still streaked their rocky fangs. Finally, we rounded a bend beside the sparkling Aparima and drove into Otautau, a typical New Zealand country town. The house we were to rent was on a hill and if we looked over the township and the fertile farmland beyond, far away to the west, we could see the roughened skyline where the last fling of the Southern Alps fractured into the wild mountains of Fiordland.

As far as first impressions went, it was a promising start.

~

In the end, the six weeks turned into twenty-seven years of active veterinary service.

Daryl Marshall had been the first vet to stay in the area for any length of time. But by the time we arrived, in 1979, he had retired from full time veterinary practice to develop a sheep and deer farm near to Otautau, and he only provided a veterinary service to a few clients of his own. His original employers were the farmers of the "Western Southland Veterinary Club" and it was they who were about to employ me. The Vet

Club system was the standard model responsible for establishing veterinary practices throughout rural New Zealand. They worked especially well by drawing vets into remote areas where they would otherwise have been unwilling to commit to the investment of setting up a practice. The farmers provided all the staff, plant and facilities necessary to run a modern veterinary practice. The farmer committee I worked with were very supportive, but the system had its frustrations and eventually I found, as Daryl had, that I wanted to run my own business. Farmers are self-reliant businessmen themselves and, in the end they relented to a proposal Daryl and I put to them, and let us lease the premises.

Daryl put a manager on his farm and the two of us set up a partnership: Marshall and Hicks Veterinary Surgeons. I couldn't have wished for a better partner. MHVS was a success from the start, no small part of which was due to Daryl's unshakeable self-belief and strong work ethic. But if Daryl worked hard, he also played hard. The partnership, with its shared after hours duty roster, had freed him from the 24/7 obligations of being a solo vet and he was better able to indulge his passion for the outdoors. When he wasn't on his farm he was hunting or fishing. Each of his forays resulted in the deaths of some poor, unfortunate creatures: deer, trout, flounder, crayfish, whitebait. Years later, as the practice grew and we employed more vets, he took a bit of teasing about this: wasn't it ironic that he should spend his weekdays saving animals' lives, but his free weekends doing the exact opposite? It was noticeable his colleagues took care not to push him too much, being keen to partake of the spoils. By this stage I had long ceased catapulting cats so I, too, occasionally indulged in this gentle ribbing. In many ways Daryl and I were poles apart, but our partnership worked because we respected each other. He was certainly less risk-averse than me, but sometimes his gambling instincts led us astray.

JC, a potential new client, and a shrewd dairy farmer, must have recognised this. Daryl came back from a visit to a sick cow enthused by JC's challenge: "John, he told me he was fed up with calling in vets who used s**tloads of expensive drugs, only to have the bloody things die on him a day or two later."

"How do you know we're going to do any better?" I asked, well aware that clients who swap vets once are quite prone to doing it again.

"Well he proposes a 'double or quits' policy. If we treat a cow and it recovers, we can charge him double fees. On the other hand, if the cow dies, he doesn't pay anything."

I detected a few loopholes in this rather loose arrangement: "And who is to police our success or failure rate?"

"He seems a genuine sort of joker. I reckon we should give it a go."

So we did. JC lived out on a limb. It was a one hundred kilometre round trip to treat his sick cows, and he certainly knew which ones to pick for veterinary attention. We soon found out that JC was a pretty competent operator who could very well manage the routine easy calvings and milk fevers, so we were left with the thin cows cast in ditches with rotten calves inside them—patently beyond the scope of the most gifted clinician with a limitless armoury of drugs at his command. It soon became apparent that the occasions when we failed, and were not able to charge, far exceeded the times when we were able to charge double. We cut our losses by not pumping "diers" with expensive drugs—a lesson all enthusiastic young vets need to learn—and before the new month started we had terminated that particular arrangement. JC seemed unconcerned; he had proved his point. From samples we had taken from some of his sick cows we revealed reason enough to account for their poor condition. By the following spring JC had corrected the selenium and copper deficiencies we had discovered and, with his cows sleeker and fatter, their productivity lifted and their death rate lessened dramatically.

Dairy cows calving in springtime are on a metabolic knife-edge. If they are thin they have no reserves, and it is frequently impossible to treat them and restore them to health. Even if they live they are unlikely to be productive animals: unlikely to milk well and unlikely to get pregnant again. JC's "double or quits" strategy had pointed us towards the correct approach—prevention is better than cure. He remained a loyal client for many years: definitely a genuine sort of joker.

~

Soon Daryl and I were joined by other vets, each with their own very different skills and personalities. Giles and Rosie Gill, husband and wife—both vets—were the first. They had graduated from Edinburgh University and worked around the world before deciding to settle in Otautau with their young family. Giles soon joined the partnership, but Rosie, with their young family, chose to work part-time. She was a consummate small animal surgeon.

Giles' father was a highly skilled engineer who had imbued his son with a reverence for all things mechanical. On his first working day at MHVS, Giles made Daryl and me fully aware that the hoof knives we had been using to pare the horn from the feet of lame cows were woefully blunt. The next day our knives came back from his workshop gleaming from a long overdue regrinding, installed in neat sheaths he had made out of hosepipe. It took a while to adjust to these re-invigorated tools. Not only did they now slice through horn like butter, but anything else that happened to be caught out by the user's follow-through. Daryl and I both returned from our rounds sporting bandaged fingers.

Not content with a practical, reliable means of transport, Giles preferred his ancient MG sports car. When she failed, as she frequently did, he would work through the night to make her roadworthy again. As a last resort he had a vintage Land Rover to fall back on, or even his three-wheeler Morgan. Farmers loved to see him turn up in one of these classic vehicles.

One of our biggest dairy farmers—part of the vanguard of the great expansion in dairying we were about to witness—had purchased over two hundred heifers that he wanted us to dehorn. Horns are a great inconvenience in large herds. Apart from the danger to people handling horned cattle, horns also inflict nasty injuries on other cows. Normally, dairy cattle are dehorned when they are only a few weeks old. It becomes a much bigger task when the animals are adult. We needed two vets to handle this job efficiently, and planned accordingly.

I duly turned up on the farm at the appointed time in my practical four-wheel drive vehicle with all the gear. It was a bit of a struggle getting to the shed, because the farmer had recently gravelled the track using large river stones. My trusty chariot lurched and scrunched up to the farmer's shed and I waited with him for Giles to appear. After a while (for some reason

Giles' mechanical bent has never applied to clocks, or if it does, he ignores them) the little green MG screamed into sight and, in a brilliant display of rallying skills, danced over the boulders and pulled up alongside us—late as usual. Pardon me for my punctuality, but it did rather stick in my craw when the farmer turned to me and commented, almost with disdain: "Now that's what I call style."

Once we got going, everything went smoothly enough. Giles risked his limbs, dextrously administering the local anaesthetic nerve block behind the eye socket of each heifer as they moved up the race and into a large headbail. I was stationed beside this to apply the guillotine-like dehorners and staunch any spouting arteries. It was a bloody and tiring afternoon.

The MG was Giles' beloved workhorse. While the rest of us just about managed to cram the copious amounts of equipment vets have to carry into our spacious station wagons, Giles travelled light—stowing all his gear in the miniscule boot of his MG. The overflow tumbled over the backseat and he was constantly forced to elbow aside his inanimate front row passengers-of-the-day. Drums of drench, an ancient leather probang, lubricants and stirrup pumps, calving jacks: all jostled for the limited space available.

Inevitably, the MG fell victim to increasingly long bouts of sick leave and, after many years of devoted service to the farming community, finally succumbed to metal fatigue and lack of replacement parts. She had been repeatedly bellied on gravel roads and pulled out of mud holes by tractors. It may have been a sad day for Giles when he finally bade her farewell, but at last her passengers were spared intimidating glimpses—through holes in the floorboards—of tar seal and road markings flashing by at mind-blurring speed. No longer were they to be frozen on winter journeys to veterinary meetings. The old jersey used as a draft excluder for the gap by the window died with the car. We placed an epitaph in our newsletter to farmers under the heading "RIP" (rust in pieces).

Giles diligently applied his mechanical skills to our business. He soon became our Mr Fixit around the clinic. As a handyman his ability was, at times, truly dazzling.

On occasions vets have to evaluate semen from rams or bulls to check that they are fertile. An infertile sire is as useful to a farmer as a tit on a skylark. Obtaining the sample can be messy and dangerous. It is one of many examples where the medical profession holds an advantage over us poor vets. A private room and a few copies of Playboy don't cut the mustard with your average bull; millions of years of evolution decree that he needs a compliant cow to "get his rocks off". However, human ingenuity knows no bounds, and bulls at AI centres can be trained to mount dummy cows and ejaculate into pre-warmed artificial vaginas. This method is impractical with untrained animals and in unsuitable facilities. Nevertheless, by some strange lateral thinking and experimentation, man or womankind has devised a way round this: rams and bulls can be electro-ejaculated. A probe with electrical leads is lubricated (vets usually have gallons of lubricant sloshing around in the back of their vehicles) and inserted into the bull's rectum. When the dial on a rheostat is twiddled, the pulsed current usually induces an unsteady, pulsing erection. This is followed, at an unpredictable interval, by a randomly directed ejaculation. It takes skill on behalf of some poor unfortunate, grovelling around underneath the bull, to track the progression of the twitching tip of the bull's penis. He or she has to catch the spurt in a polystyrene receptacle. It is important to avoid touching the glans—polystyrene on the delicate mucus membrane seems to be a big turn-off—and to avoid receiving a full facial "cum shot". The semen sample is then checked under a microscope.

The early days of the deer industry produced many challenges as farmers and vets sorted out what facilities were required to handle these flighty animals. Stags in the "roar", when they are ready to mate, are notoriously dangerous, yet one of our farmers wanted to find out whether his $12,000 elk stag, Armageddon (not his real name), was fertile. The most practical method of collecting Armageddon's semen appeared to be by electro-ejaculating him, but for the safety of all concerned it would have to be under heavy sedation. It is important that the electrical contacts on the probe are in close contact with the rectal lining. Our ram probe was too small, and the bull probe, very likely, too big. We needed a probe of intermediate size. None seemed to be available commercially: despite checking through all available back numbers of *Health Pride*, looking alternately under "stag probe" or "electro-ejaculation", we were unable to find what we were looking for. Perhaps, being crude vets, we were too direct; possibly the item was there, displayed by some towel-clad model to demonstrate how to electro-stimulate away "those tired-looking bags under your eyes". What were we to do?

Daryl and I were enormously impressed when, next morning, Giles arrived at work with a stag probe—testament to a night of meticulous wood and metal craftsmanship, and a smidgen of electronic wizardry. A few hours later Armageddon was stretched out on the floor under a heavy dose of "Fentaz". The stag probe performed to perfection. A good semen sample was obtained and, little though Armageddon may have appreciated his good luck, he was spared execution and able to spend another season with his hinds.

~

My detailed descriptions of such procedures may seem gratuitous, but the majority of a farm vets' time is spent manipulating animal genitalia. The profitability of most farming enterprises is linked to the fertility and fecundity of their livestock. Perhaps, in my frankness, I have shaken the cherished delusions of tender-hearted romantics about life as a country vet. However, part of the conditioning of young veterinary students involves erasing inhibitions about hitherto taboo topics. A typical example would be our first ventures into the bowels of man's most stoical friend… the cow.

Chapter Ten

Fertility in Beast and Man

The turtle lives 'twixt plated decks
Which practically conceal its sex.
I think it clever of the turtle
In such a fix to be so fertile. – Ogden Nash

At last, in my fourth year at university, we were getting to grips with animals in genuine clinical situations. We clambered into the university vans in small enthusiastic teams and visited farms where we learned how to rope lame cows so that we could examine their feet, performed caesarean sections, and practised rectal examinations.

The first time I put my hand up a cow's backside I was immediately aware of the alarming clamping power of her anal sphincter. She resented my intrusion and was keen to expel the offending arm. My hand floated ineffectually around what could well have been a bag of warm porridge. Of course it wasn't porridge, a fact which was brought home to me when she coughed. It was an effective manoeuvre on her part. It brought my little rectal foray to an untimely end, and spattered my face with hot shit—much to the amusement of the onlookers. I had "lost face" in front of them in a manner far too literal for my liking. What's more, the cervix, uterus and ovaries, which I was supposed to locate and assess through the wall of her rectum, had totally evaded my cautious efforts to find them. I was aware that if you are too rough there is a risk of your fingers going through the rectal wall and inducing a fatal peritonitis; although we had been told that the chance of this happening is far less in cows than in mares. But how rough is too rough?

The cows were lined up in their stalls, each with an attendant student. The tutor passed behind the row of rectal rookies, all studiously intent on acquiring this essential skill of bovine medicine.

"What did you find, Hardcastle?" he asked my neighbour.

"The right ovary was larger than the left, sir. I think there is a corpus luteum on it, and there seems to be a follicle developing on the left ovary."

"Very good, Hardcastle. She was reported cycling about two weeks ago, which is consistent with what you've found." And, turning to me, noticing my soiled countenance, he advised me to "go with the flow". "Don't leave your hand in the rectum if she starts to strain. Let your hand slide out and, when she's finished, gently reinsert it again. Have another try."

But my cow was an old trooper fed up with the attentions of inexperienced students. When I re-inserted my hand she ballooned her rectum. All I could feel was a taut rectal wall. There are means to get round that, too. I refrained from asking Hardcastle because he would probably know and, right at that moment, I felt more inclined to murder him.

It wasn't until I started my first job in New Zealand and had been in an intensive dairy practice in Taranaki for several months that I finally felt confident about the process. I owed this to the patient supervision of Hank de Jong, my first boss. By the time I had completed a season there I truly felt that I could "see" with my finger tips and determine the stage of pregnancy of a cow to within tolerable limits, distinguish a mummified foetus from a healthy one, or establish whether the cow was actually cycling or had stopped and become anoestrus (literally, "without heat").

The casual observer might well wonder why farm vetting seems so intrinsically linked to the rectal examination of cattle. Why have vets always got one hand inserted up a cow's backside? The answer relates to fertility. It may seem obvious, but is sometimes forgotten, that cows need to get pregnant in order to milk. For the dairy farmer, no milk equals no income. If a cow is going to keep milking, she needs to get pregnant once a year. There are a mass of mathematical possibilities and limitations.

A cow's pregnancy lasts roughly 285 days. There are 365 days in the year so, unless she is going to calve later next year, she needs to get pregnant within 80 days of giving birth. Depending on her age and health and any difficulties she has around calving time she won't be on heat and ready to mate till at least 42 days after giving birth, and from then on she'll come on heat (cycle) at 21 day intervals. But, on average, she'll need to be mated 1.5 times to conceive. Furthermore, 5% of pregnancies are naturally incompatible and are aborted. The odds really are stacked against the average New Zealand dairy farmer striving to have all his cows calved in spring and ready to be mated again before Christmas. He needs all the help he can from those tired vets as they plunge their arms into cow after cow.

"Could I have a vet out at tomorrow morning's milking to check 300 cows? They've calved more than six weeks but haven't yet cycled." In October and November the day books of New Zealand vets are filled with such requests. Sometimes it would be nice to go back to those days as a struggling university student when our tutor gave us useful tips: "As you will have noticed, rectal palpations are quite tiring. It would be unrealistic to be expected to do more than ten to a dozen such examinations at any one time."

Ever expanding herds have certainly pushed New Zealand vets well past these boundaries. On the other hand, the number of vets with OOS, elbow, shoulder and back injuries is becoming quite alarming. This work falls on the fewer and fewer experienced vets still willing to do it, as a new generation of veterinary graduates, selected for their training solely on the basis of academic ability, shun the rural lifestyle and the immense physical demands of dairy practice.

In the early seventies, when we dealt with non-cycling cattle, we were far less sophisticated in our approach. Cows, as we have seen, have a period in their cycle when they are "on heat"—every 3 weeks. Heat lasts from a matter of hours, to a couple of days—depending on the time of year. It is only when they come on heat that they are sexually receptive, about to ovulate, and able to conceive. Hormones control the whole process. The hormones that induce animals to come on heat, or oestrus, are known as oestrogens. In my early days in practice, diethylstilboestrol (DES), a synthetic oestrogen, was widely used as an injection for cows both to prevent conception—as when a bull mismated a line of heifers—or to induce cows which weren't cycling to come on heat, so that they could be mated. DES was also used as a growth promotant in meat producing animals.

Farmers and vets loved DES. Within a few days of the injections, the cows would be riding each other and "bulling" like mad. They were on heat. There was only one problem: although they manifested all the outward signs of sexual receptivity, and could be mated, the matings were infertile because they were not ovulating. DES only did half the job. However, the hope was that the treated cows would be "jolted" into performing properly and their subsequent heats would be fertile. Sometimes it seemed to work, but there again, "tickling the ovaries"—the mere act of palpating them—also seemed to help. In truth, given time, most well fed cows will start cycling again after calving; it's just that under modern farming systems time is money and feed is sometimes short. Most farmers haven't the patience to wait.

These days there is a far more complete understanding of the complexities of bovine reproduction, and subtler and less harmful drugs have been developed to treat infertility. DES, the drug that my generation of cow vets splashed around with gay abandon, has been banned. It has been identified as a human carcinogen capable of causing uterine cancer in women, and even in the children of women who have been exposed to it.

If I revisit that early scene where, with varying degrees of confidence, we palpated the ovaries of cattle, I am reminded how much of what we then accepted as fact was, in the light of later revelations, grossly erroneous. Whilst it is possible to identify corpora lutea on the ovaries of cattle by palpation, it has been shown that even experienced operators will miss a large percentage of them. The significance that can be attached to finding a follicle on an ovary has changed completely because we now understand that cows have waves of follicles, sometimes two or three per cycle and not every one is destined to burst and release an egg down the fallopian tube ready for fertilisation. Yet for years some high-powered veterinary practices had indulged in an orgy of "ovary scoring" each spring, categorising the supposed degree of infertility for each cow, computerising the records and allocating

94

individual fertility treatments to each one. These technocrats dismissed those of us who disputed the relevance of such procedures. Surveys have also shown that all those vets who assuredly claimed to be able to detect intra-uterine infections by palpation, or by the even more painstaking procedure of checking each cow visually with a vaginal speculum, were only picking up a fraction of the cows affected.

The greatest changes in our management of infertility have come from an acknowledgement of the role of good nutrition and the importance of breeding from fertile stock. In the long run, it is not a good policy to breed from sub-fertile animals that have been induced to conceive by chemical interventions. So saying, I condemn Viv and myself as a breeding pair. We should have been culled long ago...

~

During the oil crisis in the 1980s the government introduced measures designed to reduce fuel consumption. The maximum speed limit for anyone anywhere was reduced to a mind-numbingly boring 80 kph. The other novelty was the "car-less" day, the one day in the week on which you elected not to use your car. As a vet, I was exempted and could use my car, even on this forbidden day, providing I was using it for veterinary work. For families in rural areas the restriction was minimal if they owned, as many did, more than one vehicle. It was then simply a matter of nominating a different weekday for each vehicle.

Unfortunately, Viv and I had only one car between us, and Viv was caught doing 85 kph as we drove to a meeting in Invercargill. It was supposed to be our car-less day, as stipulated by the sticker displayed prominently on our windscreen. The meeting was held infrequently, and we knew we would either have to break the law to attend it or go through the prolonged procedure of applying for an exemption. What would be the penalty for two transgressions in one hit?

The traffic cop peered through the windows of our little Mazda, as though looking for contraband. The back was piled to the gunnels with stomach tubes, cartons of drugs, lubricant and all the other accoutrements required of a country vet. It was a pain to unload them just for a trip into town. "I suppose you're rushing to an urgent veterinary job." The excuse was being offered to Viv on a plate.

"No," answered my honest wife, "We're on our way to Invercargill. My husband's got the day off and we have no other means of getting to an important meeting".

"All right… I'll let you off this time for being honest." His cheerful response seemed to augur well for the rest of the day.

The meeting to which Viv and I were hurrying was about adoption. After several years of trying to conceive, and undergoing the usual undignified and painful gamut of tests, we had at last come to the decision that if we ever wanted children, we would have to adopt them. At the meeting we began to appreciate the difficulties that lay ahead. Quite rightly, the government adoption agency assesses the needs of the children first. If they can be placed in the tried and tested environment of an already happy family, they are. Infertile couples who have no children are carefully assessed for suitability and put on a list. We settled in for a long and uncertain wait and, to break the tension, took off on a tramping holiday in the Southern Alps.

We were lucky. After only a few weeks we strongly suspected that Viv was pregnant, but how many times had our false hopes been dashed? However, this time the tests seemed to support our hunch. It is beyond me to describe the joy of the first ultrasound scan where we could see that Viv was, indeed, pregnant. It brought tears to our eyes. More amazingly, this miraculous new technology could accurately age our little spark of life. We deduced that our child was conceived on an Alpine herbfield surrounded by snowy peaks. The love of such places certainly seems to have infused her blood; Emily has always loved the great outdoors.

All true scientists will abjure this thesis. The setting in which a conception occurs cannot, of course, influence the personality of the resulting child, any more than a pregnant woman seeing a hare may cause her child to be born with a hare lip. The first is a notion of poesy, the second, of superstition. The science of human fertility is as wrapped in psychology as it is in physiology. What was the rationale behind the years of infertility Viv and I had suffered? Such episodes— whereby an infertile couple conceive just when they've given up trying—are not uncommon. It serves to illustrate how much our minds influence our bodies.

Luckily, for Viv and me our barrier to fertility was broken with Emily's birth. We did not have to wait long for our second daughter, Morwenna, to complete our precious family.

Chapter Eleven

Naughtie Herbs

Poison is in everything, and no thing is without poison. The dosage makes it either a poison or a remedy. – Paracelsus

New Zealand was a benign land for settlers: no snakes and only one rare and slightly venomous spider—the katipo. The giant Harpagornis eagle had been the only large predator. Its talons may have been as large as a tiger's paw, but it faded to extinction once its food source—the meaty, flightless moa—was hunted to oblivion by early Maori. With a few exceptions even the plants are benign. The early European settlers deplored the sharp-leaved spear grasses ("Spaniards") that stabbed them and their horses as they rode across the tussock plains. These plants are still bothersome and can leave festering wounds on dogs working sheep in rough country. The xenophobia of the early colonists is revealed in the names they gave these less desirable plants, such as "Horrid Spaniard" (*Aciphylla horrida*) and "Giant Spaniard" which forms huge clumps up to three metres tall. On dry banks and slopes the back-country is also stoutly defended by the spiny "Wild Irishman" in dense, perverse thickets—now more commonly known by its onomatopoeic Maori name— "Matagouri". More formidable still is the "Fierce Nettle" (*Urtica ferox*)—a woody shrub far more dangerous than any nettles the early settlers would have encountered in their home countries. Fatal poisoning in man has been recorded and, as a piece of veterinary esoterica, it is on record that the extract from just five stings can kill a guinea pig. However, by and large, the flora of New Zealand held few dreads. There are very few poisonous plants.

For a vet, this is a bit disappointing. Plant poisonings of livestock make an interesting diversion from the routine of pregnancy testing cattle, palpating rams testicles or trimming cows' feet.

There is, however, one conspicuously poisonous family of plants, the *Coriariaceae*. Even for the most ardent classicist, this is a bit of a mouthful. Not surprisingly, the Maori name "Tutu" is preferred. The pioneering farmers were probably not much "into" classical ballet, so this would not have caused them confusion but, being Kiwis, and not averse to butchering Maori words, they abbreviated the name further and, amongst farmers at least, it is now almost universally known as "Toot".

The early settlers lost large numbers of animals to Toot poisoning. All parts of the plant are poisonous except for the flesh of the fruit. Within the fruit, however, there are fine seeds, which are poisonous. So, although the Maoris made a drink from the fruit and the settlers compounded a wine, there was some risk attached to the process. Canon Stack related an incident during one of his travels with Bishop Harper in the mid 1800s. Shortly after they swallowed the wine, ...*the Canon lost all feeling in his extremities, and could scarcely retain his seat, but felt that he must fall forward on his face. A mist appeared to come over the room, and he perceived that he was being poisoned, and must ask for an emetic. Soon, however, his feet began to tingle, and the strange sensation passed. The good Bishop was similarly affected, so, judging from this case, the beverage can scarcely be recommended for general use.*

There is no antidote. Our two reverends were lucky not to be subjected to the treatment given to Maori children poisoned after eating the berries, which was to smoke them over a fire of green boughs while they were constantly shaken. Even worse was the treatment favoured by stockmen: to bleed poisoned animals by cutting a cross in the roof of the mouth. Folk memories linger, and for the want of any effective treatment, this trick is still occasionally used. There is no scientific justification for it, except that it gives anxious stockmen something to do, and some animals will recover anyway—cases of "in spite of", rather than "because of", treatment. I wonder if some of these bush surgeons would be impressed if, when they rushed their poisoned child into hospital, the physician resorted to the same barbarity.

As with most plant poisonings, the symptoms are not very specific: excitability, convulsions, coma and death. The poisonous principle is a glycoside called *tutin*. I like this aspect of plant toxicology. Most plant toxins are either glycosides or alkaloids and usually little is known about them. With a little ingenuity it is possible to invent an erudite answer to those who wish to test your knowledge of plant poisons, merely by applying a little school-boy Latin. Hence the poisonous principle of Ragwort (*Senecio jacobea*), is *jacobine*; of Hemlock (*Conium maculatum*), *coniine*; of Yew (*Taxus bacata*), *taxine*. The new wave of European immigrants to Aotearoa brought these poisonous plants with them: either by accident, in contaminated pasture seed; or deliberately, as garden plants. One of the commonest causes of animal plant poisonings occurs when stock stray into gardens, or eat clippings carelessly flung over a fence. Rhododendron, laburnum, pieris, foxglove and aconite are all common introduced plants of deadly beauty.

My first encounter with a plant poison was a personal one, as a child. It involved laburnum, a plant so poisonous that throwing a stick of laburnum for your dog can prove fatal to it. In which case "All right Fido, just one last game" would become an accurate prophesy. I plead forgiveness for my ignorance of toxicology—I was only about five years old at the time—however, I must have been an observant child because I noticed the beautiful little "pills" in their neat seed pods under the laburnum tree in our Liverpool garden…

Children's play often models itself on adult behaviour so, when we had finished killing each other ("Cowboys and Indians" being our unsophisticated vehicle for this indulgence), we sat down for a pretend dinner party under the shade of the tree. That's when we commenced 'popping' the pills. The rest is a bit hazy. I remember vomiting and crawling to the house to raise the alarm. We all survived, but we were very lucky. Laburnum is the commonest plant poison causing death in children in Britain. What a great idea to bring it to New Zealand!

Within a given plant species the concentration of toxic chemicals may also vary between plant populations, and can be influenced by variables such as the age of the plant, the soil type or the climate. Hemlock is a classic example; or, if you prefer, an example from classical times. It was supposedly an extract of hemlock that was used to execute Socrates in 399 B.C. Since the toxic effects include vomiting, incoordination and convulsions and occur 'within a few hours of ingestion' his death may not have been the dignified and serene departure described by Plato: …

and he walked about until, as he said, his legs began to fail, and then he lay on his back, according to the directions. And the man who gave him the poison now and then looked at his feet and legs; and after a while he pressed his foot hard, and asked him if he could feel; and he said, No; and then his leg, and so upwards and upwards and showed us that he was cold and stiff. And he felt then himself and said: When the poison reaches the heart, that will be the end. He was beginning to grow cold about the groin, when he uncovered his face, for he had covered himself up, and said (they were his last words) – he said: Crito, I owe a cock to Asclepius; will you remember to pay the debt? The debt shall be paid, said Crito; is there anything else? There was no answer to this question; but in a minute or two a movement was heard, and the attendants un-covered him; his eyes were set, and Crito closed his eyes and mouth. Such was the end, Echecrates, of our friend, whom I may truly call the wisest, most just, and best of all men whom I have ever known.

Plato's description of creeping paralysis has a ring of authenticity, it matches other descriptions of the end stage of hemlock poisoning when the alkaloids paralyse the motor nerve endings and depress the central nervous system. Plato, it seems, for reasons of artistic licence, left out the initial vomiting and convulsions. The splatter deaths and gore of Hollywood would have been anathema to the Greeks whose art required that scenes of death and suffering should be dignified by beauty.

Hemlock is common in New Zealand, and poisoning of livestock does occur, but not as commonly as would be expected. I have seen cattle snatching at plants on their way to a milking shed without obvious side-effects—so maybe we are fortunate and our plants contain less of the alkaloids that make this such a dangerous plant in other countries. This variability is perhaps why hemlock came to be regarded as unreliable for medicinal purposes, or as one early herbal described it, *a naughtie and dangerous herb*, and its use as such was discontinued in the nineteenth century.

Of course, many highly toxic plants have yielded useful drugs. In 1785, William Withering deduced that of the twenty ingredients in a secret family recipe to treat swollen legs (a manifestation of heart failure in humans that is rarely seen in animals), the effective element was foxglove. In the distant past of my veterinary training the most widely used drug for heart problems, usually in dogs, was digitalis—an extract from *Digitalis purpurea*, the common foxglove. Leaves of this poisonous plant floated mystically in glass-stoppered jars in the dusty dispensaries of a previous generation of pharmacists as *Tincture of digitalis*. Unfortunately, the amount of digitalis required to produce a clinically useful response in the heart muscle is close to the toxic level which induces nausea and vomiting. The trick was to hospitalise the dog for observation, and increase the daily dose until the dog started vomiting. The dose was then cut back slightly, to a level where there was no nausea. The whole process was referred to as *digitalisation*—a word that has rather different connotations today.

Alas, in veterinary medicine, we do not have the benefit of feedback from our patients about the effects of the drugs we give them. One man, on drinking tea made from foxglove leaves, became weak, nauseous and noticed yellow haloes around objects. This record, from Guy's Hospital in London, has led to speculation that digitalis poisoning affected Van Gogh's later paintings which feature haloes and a predominance of yellow. Twice he painted his physician holding a foxglove plant. If your dog is seeing yellow and painting haloes, my advice would be to consult a psychiatrist before he cuts off his ear.

More predictable synthetic derivatives of digitalis still have a place in modern medicine, but other families of even more potent cardiac drugs have largely superseded even these.

Pixie, our tireless Fox Terrier, was getting grey about the gills and finally slowing down. She had made a major contribution to the up-bringing of our daughters, as family pets do, but she was becoming increasingly breathless. Chasing games, that once seemed endless for the human participants, were finishing with a sulk after a couple of throws. She only fired into life if she spied a cat on her territory and, even then, after the initial, frantic pursuit, her enthusiasm for the post-chase, tail-up, victory patrols of her boundaries waned, and she would retire wearily to her window seat. She coughed, particularly at night, occasionally bringing up small amounts of froth. These are all classic signs of heart failure and I could clearly discern a murmur when I applied my stethoscope to her chest. Later we were able to see the cause with an ultrasound scanner: a lump on one of her heart valves. Her heart was no longer the efficient pump it should have been and, as a result of poor circulation, her lungs were becoming waterlogged.

The ideal solution for Pixie would have been to replace her defective heart valve—a matter of routine in human surgery, but scarcely economic for a family pet. Realistically, vets can only offer drugs to alleviate the symptoms.

Fortunately there are newer drugs, safer than digitalis. One category (ACE inhibitors) reduces the worst side effects of fluid accumulation. They gave

Pixie a new lease of life. Although her heart still sounded like an old washing machine, her coughing all but vanished. She perked up considerably, and had a great quality of life for another three years thanks to the little pill we ground onto her food once a day. We tried to dampen her newly re-kindled enthusiasm for chasing cats, fearing it would be her undoing, but we were never able to reverse her psychological conditioning.

~

The idea of going back to nature and using natural remedies may have romantic appeal, but applying scientific principles to isolate the active ingredients and then modify and test them to maximise efficacy and safety is surely the way to go. It is more reliable, and safer, to take an asprin for a headache than to quaff a decoction of willow bark. Both contain the active anti-inflammatory, *salicylic acid*, but herbal remedies are always going to be less reliable because of the unpredictable concentrations of their active ingredients and the risk of cross-reactions with other toxic chemicals they contain.

An example of the misuse of "natural" products is the fad to use tea tree (*Melaleuca*) oil for skin infections. It has antiseptic properties, but is toxic if ingested. There have been fatalities in cats and kittens following flea treatment with the oil. Yet parents risk it on their children. A recent report in the veterinary press described a dog which became uncoordinated, developed muscle tremors and was unable to walk for several hours after the oil was applied by its owners to treat a skin infection. Fortunately it recovered with supportive treatment. I fully agree with the conclusion of the vet who treated that dog: *The public is eager to use 'natural products' without any testing for toxicity, let alone efficacy. The lesson here is obviously not to assume that all things natural are without dangers.*

Good examples of this are *caffeine* and *nicotine*—both plant alkaloids, both natural. The dangers of excessive coffee binging and cigarettes are well known.

Another interesting plant alkaloid is *atropine*. Its source is deadly nightshade (*Atropa bella-donna*). Atropine is widely used in ophthalmology to dilate the pupil of the eye and facilitate examination of the retina at the back of the eye. An ingenious test to diagnose deadly nightshade poisoning is to put a few drops of urine from a patient suspected of being poisoned into the eye of another animal, whose pupil will, apparently, dilate fully within 30 minutes, even in bright light. To the early physicians, who diagnosed diabetes mellitus by tasting the sweetness of their patient's urine, this would have been a tame test, indeed.

Dilated pupils signify interest and, possibly, desire. To be the object of desire, however subliminally, puts the recipient under Aphrodite's spell. *Bella donna* means "beautiful lady". Historically, Italian women, bent on seduction, instilled their eyes with extract of deadly nightshade. This strategy was not without danger. The classic signs of deadly nightshade overdose are decidedly un-erotic: fever, flushing, dry mouth, blurred vision and hallucinations or, from the mnemonic countless medical students should remember: *hot as a hare, red as a beet, dry as a bone, blind as a bat and mad as a hatter.*

However, there is a far more insidious poison—also used as a cosmetic in historical times—which remains a common cause of poisoning in man and his animals today; and it is truly a trap for the unwary vet.

Chapter Twelve

An Ancient Toxin

A handful of calves sat around the pen. "What's wrong with them, Tony?" I asked.

"Ah don't reetly know. One's died and the rest won't eat or drink".

The unusual insertion of the word "rightly" and the way he pronounced it, defined Tony's origins. He had emigrated as a young man from the wilds of Derbyshire to the West Coast; but now he and his wife had bought a small dairy farm in Western Southland.

It was my first visit to his farm and I had one factor in my favour. There sometimes seems to be a subliminal trust placed by clients on vets who share their origin or ethnicity. I'm sure that a proportion of our clients preferred to see a "fair dinkum" Kiwi vet, such as Daryl, on their farm rather than a Pom like Giles or me. I milked this advantage: briefly implying a deep knowledge of all things Derbyshire. I had heard of Buxton and been down the Blue John Cave as a child. I could even have played the Derbyshire card a bit stronger and talked of Isaac Walton and *The Compleat Angler*, but that would have been pushing my luck.

After this successful meet and greet session it was axiomatic that Tony expected great things of me. The calves, however, were proving to be a big stumbling block. The more I questioned him about them, the more puzzling the case appeared. My specially favoured status, in Tony's eyes, seemed under threat.

At first sight you would not have picked that there was anything amiss with Tony's calves. I needed to examine them more closely. I stepped into the pen with a thermometer at the ready, a stethoscope round my neck and a few plastic gloves in my pockets. Ninety per cent of the illnesses vets see in calves of this age involve enteric infections—scours. Avid followers of TV documentaries about beautiful young vets' encounters with doe-eyed calves will have been misled about this. TV directors are obviously well aware that enteritis in calves, in glorious Technicolor, is not a welcome televisual feast for viewers. But Tony's calves would have been easy to film. They sat in their clean pen and did nothing. Even when I climbed in among them, they hardly stirred. Healthy calves would have been up and bunting me, looking for milk. These calves couldn't do that. They were deaf and blind—not that this was obvious from a brief glance. Their eyes looked normal, but they didn't blink or respond when something was waved in their faces.

Even before I'd examined the calves properly, Tony was applying the pressure. "I don't suppose you know what it is, then?" I was tempted to use a word I had chanced upon at some stage in my studies, a fatuous diagnosis—*amaurosis*—a blindness of unknown origin. But why blind him with science? There was more than enough blindness in that barn already.

When confronted with a novel set of symptoms, it is useful to try and pin down which body system is involved. The lack of diarrhoea around the calves ruled out a primary involvement of the alimentary system. If anything they were slightly constipated, so my plastic gloves remained in my pocket. Time to brandish my thermometer. Thermometers provide thinking time. While the farmer keeps asking him what he thinks it is, it is the vet's task to concentrate and carefully scrutinize his thermometer. If he is older, and has acquired the skill, he may even furrow his brow. At this stage it is important to remember the purpose of the furrow. It is there to inspire confidence. The vet must take care not to tip it into the realms of the *furrow-of-worry* or, even, the *furrow-of-alarm*. If the correct balance has been achieved the caring clinician will convey the semblance of being deep in thought, and that he is not to be disturbed. Great things are stirring behind that careworn forehead.

If, like me, this is the first lot of calves he has ever seen with these presenting signs, he'll be thinking something like: What the f*** makes calves suddenly go deaf and blind? If he is confident, he will discard all thoughts about his last visit here when he did a caesarean and the cow died half-an-hour after he left the farm—and its corollary: so he can't afford to stuff up this time.

Despite my brain wracking ploys, I had yet to come up with an answer.

Tony, naturally enough, was concerned about the cost; he kept banging on about how much the calves were worth. I hadn't even made a diagnosis and he wanted to know if I had something to get them better. My *do-not-disturb furrow* had not been read; besides, the temperatures of the first two calves were normal. I would have to resort to the stethoscope trick. Stethoscopes are much more useful than thermometers in such situations. The ears are physically blocked, and although I could still hear Tony's muffled burblings, I had a good excuse not to be able to render them intelligible, and I could legitimately gaze into the middle distance and strain to catch every significant nuance of bovine cardiac and respiratory pathology. I expected none. There was none. Eventually a calmer voice from my clinical training pricked through: central nervous system [CNS] involvement, afebrile and bilaterally symmetrical—these calves aren't circling or head tilting—so this is unlikely to be an infection. Could be a CNS toxin. Yes, but what? Well, what is the commonest CNS toxin on farms? And so I started thinking about lead poisoning.

Lead poisoning in livestock used to be very common on farms. Classical sources were old car batteries left lying around, or old paint tins. Lead-based paints haven't been used for years, but corrugated iron sheds painted with them abound. Sheets of tin from dismantled sheds make handy pens for calves. But Tony had raised many batches of calves through these pens over previous years and never had anything like this happen before. I scrutinised the walls of the pens and found the evidence I was looking for. The calves in this batch had definitely started to lick them. We could see where their rough tongues had taken the paint off— right down to the bare metal. It just takes one curious calf to start and the rest copy. Could this be a case of lead poisoning? I had never seen lead poisoning in calves before and at the back of my mind were the textbook descriptions of the clinical signs—and they didn't tie in at all. *Frenzy, maniacal excitement, bellowing, staggering, convulsions, head pressing, attempts to climb walls or even to attack people*: these were all text book descriptions of what to expect in cattle with lead poisoning. But the fascinating thing with so many poisonings, as we have seen, is the variability of symptoms. As with statistics, look hard enough and you will find a source to back you up. Sure enough, one book suggested that the neurological signs could manifest as either excitation or depression.

The rest of the calves slowly recovered with the expensive chelation therapy I started, even before we had laboratory confirmation of the cause. The chelating agent binds to lead and allows the body to excrete it in an inert form. I had no choice but to act immediately on my hunch since laboratory analyses can take several days, by which stage more of the calves would have died. Eventually, confirmation of my diagnosis arrived. There were abnormally high levels of lead in the kidney I had submitted from the dead calf, and the source was undoubtedly the paint—further tests proving that this was lead based. My reputation was saved.

Subsequently we saw several cases of lead poisoning in calves on other farms from ingesting lead paint, and all presented with similar signs to Tony's.

We had another perplexing case of lead poisoning, this time in dogs: two out of four dogs on a farm had stopped eating and were losing condition. Their presenting signs only partially tallied with the classic picture, as tersely described in one textbook: *Dog: May be found dead. Abdominal pain. Vomiting. Diarrhoea or constipation. Anorexia. Loss of condition. Blindness. Paralysis. Convulsions. Barking fits. Death within minutes to weeks.* It was the clinical history that alerted me: close questioning established that the dogs' kennels had been recently reconstructed from old, painted, timber. The penny dropped. A blood test confirmed our suspicions. The dog that pulled his food out of his bowl and then scoffed it off the floor was worse affected than his companion, who ate mostly from his bowl. Good table manners bring their rewards:

Lead is a cumulative poison; once it's in the body it is only slowly eliminated. Ingestion of small amounts of lead over many days obviously results in a far less dramatic set of symptoms than those from a sudden large intake but, either way, if left untreated, the end result is death.

The wonder is that it took so long for mankind to discover this. The association between lead and poisoning is a relatively recent discovery. Two thousand years ago, Latin *plumbarii* (lead workers) plied their trade with this useful metal, unaware of the danger that may have contributed to the collapse of their civilisation. There were even lead mines near Buxton, though I never got round to discussing this with Tony.

In the sixteenth century Elizabeth I popularised the use of lead as a cosmetic. Lead carbonate powder mixed in various ways with additives, such as egg whites and vinegar, was slapped onto ladies' faces as frequently as Pond's Cold Cream by our mothers' generation. It conferred that interesting pale look to its wearer. However, lead *was* known to damage the skin and, later on, it became fashionable to cover up the resulting craters and eruptions with black patches. It is hard to break people of dangerous habits, and it took over two hundred years before lead carbonate was finally replaced by zinc oxide as a skin whitening agent.

In many situations, lead is inert and benign. Its very stability in neutral conditions made it safe for routine house plumbing. The main concern for local authorities came with pollution and acid rain late in the last century. In acid conditions lead slowly dissolves. Any lead which is ingested is very effectively absorbed from the acid environment of our stomachs. Once it has been absorbed, it is not readily excreted from the body. Minute amounts slowly build up, interfering with the complex biochemistry of life: clogging up those Krebs' cycle enzymes.

Conversely, large lumps of lead in the form of bullets or shotgun pellets can remain harmlessly inert in the more neutral tissues of our bodies for years. Many war veterans harbour shrapnel in various parts of their anatomy with no risk of lead poisoning. Vets quite commonly find shotgun pellets peppering the hindquarters of gundogs that may have been x-rayed for an entirely different reason. Generally speaking, they are best left alone—an observation that perhaps goes for the patients' owners as well.

Chronic low-level ingestion of lead was linked with high levels of juvenile delinquency in British cities. Unfortunately the progressive removal of lead from plumbing and motor fuels does not seem to have resulted in any general improvement in behaviour. I had a well-leaded Liverpudlian childhood, along with millions of other Brits. I am the product of a lead-plumbed house. I quaffed the leaded petrol fumes from a thousand car exhausts as I cycled to school each day. But perhaps I was lucky, for mine was a privileged childhood, I was never forced to eat my meals off the linoleum (another lead-containing product) and, in my humble opinion, I have yet to make the transition from eccentricity into barking madness.

~

Daryl had the privilege of a clean-and-green Kiwi upbringing in New Zealand's unspoilt air. Only Giles shared a background as polluted as mine. He had emerged, relatively unscathed, from the ghastly "Black Country" of the English Midlands—so named in reference to the many coalmines and slagheaps that despoil the countryside of his childhood. By contrast, Rosie came from the distilled purity of the Scottish

Highlands; no British vet could claim a less tainted background.

Sid, the vet who was about to join us, had entirely different origins, and he was bringing his family from a land of many dangers.

Chapter Thirteen

The Reluctant Immigrant

A great emigration necessarily implies unhappiness of some kind or other in the country that is deserted. – Thomas Malthus

In his few moments of relaxation at work, Daryl was challenged by the bewildering eccentricity of our tearoom chatter. He was outnumbered by Poms. Being a straightforward Kiwi the pedantry and puns eluded him at first. But the cultural mix of our practice was about to become even more diverse.

In the 1990s the dairy industry was expanding into Southland, and there was a shortage of endemic vets with the requisite skills or inclination to service it. Daryl was an exception, because other New Zealand vets seemed to have an aversion to working in the Deep South. We were forced to recruit from abroad. Fortunately, there were still overseas vets with an interest in farm animals who, owing to depressed rural economies—particularly in Britain—were eager to work anywhere in New Zealand. Many also came from South Africa. That is where we acquired our fourth partner. Marshall and Hicks was no longer an apt name and, in a fit of pragmatism, we renamed the expanded practice Otautau Vets Ltd (OVL).

For Sid, his wife and their four children, all under the age of five, the decision to emigrate must have been heartbreaking. Rather than leaving their country of birth by choice, they felt compelled to move, for the safety of their young family. Though Sid enjoyed the more serene political environment of New Zealand, there

115

were some aspects of his new career that he found less appealing.

Veterinary life in New Zealand lacks the drama of Africa's. A pathological sword of Damocles hangs over every man and beast in that vast continent. Vets and their clients in South Africa face a far greater range of virulent viral diseases, bothersome bacteria, remorseless energy-sapping parasites, perfidious pests and predators and, yes—potent poisonous plants. A vet can have real fun in South Africa dealing with dramatic deaths, mysterious maladies and exotic epidemics. Life for a vet in New Zealand, after the drama of Africa, could seem colourless and bland. Sid's anecdotes certainly added diversity to our tearoom conversations.

The corollary is that South African vets are widely respected for the excellent standard of their university qualifications and their practical abilities. We listened as Sid spoke of rinderpest and bluetongue, biliary and baboon attacks, jaagsiekte and weidektankheit. We tried hard to impress him with the longer and more complicated versions of clinical syndromes we had seen, "Remember that case of pulmonary hypertrophic osteoarthropathy we saw in that hind last week, Giles?" But for everything we had seen, Sid had seen it too, usually with knobs on—not as a matter of show, he really had—and his skills were highly valued by us. He added another dimension to our team.

Being bilingual in English and Afrikaans would not appear to be an asset in Southland, but on occasions it was. Entrepreneurial dairy farmers seeking cheap land were flowing into the province and gradually displacing long-established sheep farming families. This was an economic blessing for an area depressed by years of poor returns to sheep farmers and, because dairy farmers use vets far more intensively than sheep farmers, it was providing a major boost to our veterinary business.

There was increasing optimism that Southland would be restored to some of its former affluence, the days when wool fetched a pound (sterling) for a pound (avoirdupois). Unfortunately, silver linings are shrouded in cloud. The carefree, sunlit days lessened. Successful entrepreneurs are hard-nosed businessmen. Assertiveness has its place, but it is not always a virtue when you are on the receiving end. A few of these new clients were unreasonably demanding.

Southland farming was being infused with new farming blood, not just from dairying areas of the North Island, but from around the world. Some Dutch dairy farmers had sold up their milk supply quotas in Holland and were able to build up sizeable herds in New Zealand on the proceeds. It took guts, skill and hard work, qualities for which their countrymen are well known. Naturally, some of them tended to import labour from their home country and though they had a good grasp of English, Dutch—to mix metaphors—was the *lingua franca* on those farms.

For all the vets, with the exception of Sid, visits to such farms gave us a good lesson about the insularity of English speakers around the world. We are generally ignorant of other languages. On farms where Dutch prevailed the tables were sometimes turned on us and we worked without the usual ribbing and yarns that make farm visits so enjoyable. Afrikaans is, basically, mediaeval Dutch; so Sid did have a fair idea of what was being said, though he didn't usually let on.

One evening Sid was called out to assist a cow that was having difficulty calving. The farmer and his worker were waiting for him at the milking shed. As he unpacked his gear he heard a comment in Dutch along

117

the lines of "Let's hope this bastard isn't as useless as the last one". Sid, knowing that the vet to whom this slur applied was both extremely experienced and competent, decided to bite his tongue.

The calf was too big and Sid had no choice but to perform a caesarean. He was going to have to listen to the conversation for a good long time. It continued in the same vein. Even for the slickest of operators, with ample assistance and good facilities, a caesarean takes between an hour and an hour-and-a-half. Sid clipped the skin and administered the local anaesthetic. Apparently this wasn't done half as well as they would have done it in Holland. Apart from a few basic instructions and requests for assistance (in English), Sid bided his time. The surgery went as well as could be expected. The farmer and his worker helped to pull a large calf from the incision in the flank and attended to it while Sid carefully stitched up the wound, repairing the uterus first and then bringing together the muscle layers and the tough skin. The cow remained standing throughout. The calf was alive and soon attempting to stand. It was a job well done, not that he expected any praise for it. The Dutch conversation had veered round to how much the owner expected to be ripped off for the vet turning out at this time of night...

Revenge is sweet. Sid gave careful instructions in clear English about the cow's after-care and supplied antibiotic injections for the following days. When he had packed his gear and was ready to drive off he casually remarked, in Afrikaans, "Goodnight gentlemen. I'll send you my account in the morning."

A splutter sounds the same in Dutch or English!

Paper work was never Sid's strong point, so his threat was empty; but the farmer wasn't to know that.

~

In the beginning Sid hid his light under a bushel. This is a wise strategy for any vet starting a new job. If you're not too careful you will land the veterinary equivalent of the new builder's apprentice being sent to purchase a left-handed hammer, or tin of striped paint. I myself had been caught out this way.

One of the first jobs I was assigned on my arrival in New Zealand followed this pattern. "John, would you mind going up to 'old man Palmer' and dehorning a couple of heifers for him?" I always looked forward to visiting the rougher farms tucked up under the gleaming cone of Mount Taranaki, right next to the National Park boundary, so I keenly assented. What nobody told me was that "old man Palmer" (OMP) would not have been out of place in the previous century. He was single and ninety-nine per cent deaf, and therefore had no use for a phone. He didn't drive. If he needed a vet for a routine matter (don't ask me what he did in an emergency) he wrote a letter. The visit would be arranged and written in the desk diary at the clinic for a few days later, allowing time for a letter of confirmation to reach OMP so that he could be ready for the vet. This also provided adequate time for all the vets "in the know" to arrange to be busy at that particular hour. Unfortunately, I wasn't in the know, and my naivety was duly rewarded.

I arrived at the farm and leaned on the rather rickety railings of the primitive yard where OMP had penned his heifers. It was relaxing in the warm spring sunshine, but there was no sign of my client. I looked up to the gleaming snows of Fantham's Peak, already receding as spring advanced, and enjoyed the sun beating on my back. Why rush? The other vets seemed to have busied themselves with the remaining calls booked in when I had left the clinic and, as far as I knew, I had no urgent claims on my time.

My reveries were interrupted by a vice-like grip clamping my arm just above the elbow and a rasping exhalation in my ear—reminiscent of the unearthly hissing made by possums squabbling at the dead of night. In those days Peter Jackson's version of Gollum was, fortunately, yet to be realised—or I would have had an immediate cardiac arrest.

OMP preferred to grasp his victim firmly. Past experience must have taught him that the first reaction of his fellow men, in the face of the overwhelming assault of his wet, noisy and olfactory attempts at communication, was to retreat. OMP had no concept of personal space. On close inspection (there was no other option) his appearance was consistent with long years of living alone. He obviously shared no living companionship save that of his own robust and flourishing micro-flora and fauna. And, generously, there seemed to be no reluctance on his part to share them with me. When he was sure he had got his message across, I was released. This took some time, because his utterances were unintelligible and I was slow to realise that it was safer to pretend I knew and nod agreeably. Immediately I was free, I opened the car boot, wiped my face with a towel, and, keeping well away from OMP, proceeded with the job in hand. Whenever I had to visit OMP again, I made sure, on arrival, to position myself where I would be safe from ambush. This was infrequently: I also took care to look ahead in the diary.

In truth, the episode was one of sadness rather than terror. OMP could not respond to the spoken word, on account of his deafness, but neither did he appear to register other cues implicit in normal communication.

Body language or facial expressions were meaningless to him, as I adjudged from his blank responses. OMP just charged around doing things his way and you had to fall in as best you could. The reality of everyday life for OMP on his lonely farm will remain an untold story, unless he has chosen to drive his trusty fountain pen across fields of quarto; but, alas, those few rough letters to Eltham Vets gave no hint of any hidden literary talent. Without communication, the mind is imprisoned within its bony walls; thoughts go round in ever diminishing circles; there is no outlet.

I'm sure Sid must have had similar experiences in South Africa. Of course, Daryl, Giles or I, being honourable men, would never have exposed him to such hazards without first warning him. However, that didn't necessarily prevent him thinking that we had contrived to do just that.

The procedure for removing the semi-soft velvet antler from stags—develveting—involves, firstly, sedating them. Once they are quietly sitting or lying on the ground it is possible to administer a local nerve block—for your sake as well as theirs you don't want them to feel pain—and, after a wait, saw off the antler. Injecting the sedative can be unnerving, particularly if the stags are large and aggressive, and especially if the pens in which you are expected to spike them with your robust, sixteen gauge needle are poorly designed. Given a choice most stags will try and avoid you by running away. A square pen permits them to do this. You can take up a central position in the pen and as they go past it is relatively safe, using a syringe on the end of a long pole, to smoothly glide the needle into a muscle. But it all takes practice.

Develveting was unfamiliar to Sid. We gave him some basic training then, soon after his arrival in

Southland, it fell upon him to develvet some large and rather stroppy hybrid elk stags on a local farm. One of the problems here was that the injection pens were long and narrow. When you approach a stag in such a pen, with your pole syringe at the ready, you are, in essence, cornering him. There are only two ways the stag can evade you—either through you or over you. If, as you start your approach, he stands there with lolling tongue and grinding teeth, discretion decrees you adopt another tactic if you want to live to fight another day. Experienced vets learn to read the body language of their patients and have a fair idea of when it is safe to proceed and when to draw back—but the boundaries are sometimes blurred, or crossed when they shouldn't be. Clambering up a seven-foot hold-less wall and balancing on the top with a loaded syringe in order to inject a stag from a position of relative safety takes much more time, but is infinitely safer than risking the shortcut. After this episode Sid was unable to complain that veterinary life in New Zealand was un-exciting. In fact, hadn't we all heard him over the radio-telephone when he arrived on the farm? "Man! I may need some help with these; they're as big as kudus!" There was no further radio contact for some time. Somehow Sid managed in the end, as we all did in those days. We didn't have the luxury of back-up vets in our small and very varied practice. If you were out in the back blocks and a call came in for a neighbouring farm, you just had to cope with whatever came your way. If a horse with colic was five minutes from you, but three-quarters of an hour's drive from the clinic, and there were no free vets, you couldn't say "but I don't do horses". However, specialisation is the way modern veterinarians are training—with scant acknowledgement of the importance of being a generalist in isolated rural areas. Nevertheless, after his encounter with the kudu-sized stags, Sid became very cautious about what he was being sent to do.

When the delightful but no-nonsense, tweed-jacketed Mrs Cavalry Twill rang to have a couple of her donkeys' feet trimmed, Sid seemed reluctant to heed her call. He confided that he didn't really know much about donkeys. I was about to pin a dog's leg, Daryl had five hundred rams against his name for blood-testing and Giles had missed his lunch and was late to pregnancy test some heifers. We were all probably secretly relieved that we did have genuine and pressing reasons not to go out to Mrs CT's donkeys, so Sid had no choice but to be "volunteered" to accept the honour. After all, we said encouragingly, it is not so very different from trimming a horse's feet. In retrospect Sid must have known, like us, that this wasn't true; but he had painted himself into a corner. Donkeys have extremely tough and elastic horn and it doesn't trim easily. Even with a Giles Gill specially sharpened hoof knife this was going to be hard work. And so it proved. Donkeys aren't always tractable. If they don't want their hooves trimmed; they tend to lean on you, which, since they are low-slung, makes for back-breaking work.

Sid returned from his task later that day. Nothing was said about his donkey visit. However, it was interesting for us to note that thereafter Mrs CT always requested that Sid attend her donkeys. I was intrigued. When, at some later date, it befell me to visit her small-holding, she raved about how knowledgeable Sid was about donkeys and how he had explained to her that there was a donkey stud on a farm neighbouring his when he was in South Africa, for which he used to do a lot of work. In light of his initial protestations of ignorance, this was, indeed, a remarkable discovery. We soon learned that Sid, while not shy of recounting his tales from South Africa, was remarkably astute about what he chose to reveal: a man who could hold his counsel if there was a risk of it leading him into trouble. Take his position on ostriches …

Just because he came from South Africa, home to ostriches, Sid informed us, it didn't mean that he had ever had anything to do with them. In fact—he was quite vehement about this—there was no way he was going to deal with them. The donkey episode led us to suspect that he knew more than he was letting on. We tried to get to the bottom of it, but argued unconvincingly. "Aren't you just burying your head in the sand over these birds, Sid? The way everyone is talking, ostriches are the future. They could be great business for us." Sid didn't even rise to the debate— beyond correcting us about the head in the sand myth ascribed to ostriches (we suspected he would).

Daryl and I both reckoned we were getting a bit long in the tooth to become involved in this latest farming fad. We had been through the goat boom, the fitch craze and seen the rise of the deer industry. Ostriches didn't really appeal to us and we doubted (correctly) that fortunes would ever be realised. And, couldn't they disembowel you with one powerful kick? However, some of our clients had ostriches and we felt obliged to offer a service to them. In an isolated rural area who else could they turn to? So it was Giles who rose to this particular, but rather short-lived challenge. Before long, he found out that if he had any questions he could always turn to Sid, who suddenly seemed to be a fount of knowledge about ostriches—but only in an advisory capacity. It was Giles again, always reluctant to concede defeat in the face of a new challenge, who took a special interest in the alpacas that have recently started appearing on a few farms. Sid's abiding interest remained firmly focused on his beloved dairy cows, which is probably just as well because they had become the economic mainstay of the practice.

~

This ethnicity thing is a rum 'un. South African emigrants, including Sid, were mortally sensitive about doing the "chicken run" from South Africa. They were not emigrants of conscience who had left an apartheid state abhorrent to them. They had waited till it looked as though the wheels would fall off the post-apartheid regime. Many were abandoning their birthplace for reasons of personal safety rather than as a matter of principled anti-racism. Who can blame them? Yet they felt the onus was on them to establish their non-racist principles. Sid came from a liberal background, and consequently he was extremely insistent to present with impeccable anti-racist credentials.

Soon after his arrival Sid's principles were tested by one of our resident rednecks. Chuck was a regular client of ours who, judging by his drawl and dress— *those* boots and *that* hat, had been dragged up in the Southern States. He was a genial, blunt man, not renowned for political correctness. However, it is certainly not a vet's job to iron out the personal irregularities of those who step through his doors. If a psychologist were to observe the clientele of any veterinary practice she would find plenty to interest her: grubby old ladies with seventeen cats, lonely widows trying to crank the last ounce of life from their dead husband's dying dog; briskly efficient professional couples toting Chihuahua child substitutes in chintzy coats, thugs with Rottweilers. As long as people like Chuck kept their white hoods in their pockets and didn't light their fiery crosses in front of our No Smoking signs, we felt obliged to care for their animals. Ours not to reason why.

When Chuck brought his gun dog in for a vaccination, we introduced him to Sid as our new vet from South Africa; and Chuck, thinking he recognised a kindred spirit in Sid, decided to tell him a joke. He only got as far as the fourth word: "There was this nigger..." at which point Sid turned on his heel and walked away. It was left to one of us to inform Chuck of the error of his ways. Later on Sid was at pains to point out to us that he did not have Afrikaans ancestry and, quite rightly, that he deplored racist attitudes.

Some of us detected a slight inconsistency in his stance when he so stoutly supported his beloved Springboks, for he was a passionate fan of a rugby team which had yet to root out some of its Broederbond affiliations. We exploited this, for Sid seemed naive when it came to ironic humour. However, in the end he, too, made the weird cultural adjustments necessary to survive smoko conversations at Otautau Vets Ltd. Before long he was enriching us with tales from the amazing land of his birth and his deep veterinary knowledge. Sid was disarmingly gullible at times yet, as we shall see, his brilliant analytical mind contributed another dimension to our practice and improved the service we could offer our clients.

It takes a mix of skills and personalities to make a good team. It is so much more fun when you can accept and laugh about your differences.

Chapter Fourteen

Warbles, Noah and the Milkshake Mixer

In fact, it [fundamentalism] *offers no real explanation of origins, but simply declares that all creatures are as they are because they were originally made by an invisible power. Not only is this 'creationist' view unconvincing, but it denies us the great gift of spiritual wonder. By contrast, contemplating the evolution of planetary life over some three billion years leaves one speechless with awe. –* Lloyd Geering

My first encounter with parasitism occurred while I was a young student completing my "farm prac." experience. It was a lazy summer afternoon. I loved helping on the farm on days like this. John Mason and I chatted as we drove his twenty-five cows from the meadow to the shippon to be milked. Swifts screamed as they skimmed across a pasture thick with shining buttercups and the antique purple of meadow cranesbill: creaming the insect-laden air. Our sleek charges ambled contentedly across the warm cobbles of the yard and into the pungent shade of the stone building. This peaceful routine was the way of life for hundreds of small farmers throughout the Yorkshire Dales.

It was my job to tie the chains round the cows' necks as they foraged eagerly for the dairy nuts in the troughs in front of them or, pressing on the nose valves, sucked in the cool water. I loved the intimacy of this contact with these gentle, powerful animals. Deep down, my desire to be a vet was not based on any intellectual considerations.

John was always keen to show me, an ignorant city lad, the intricacies of his world. "Have a look at this, John," he said, nonchalantly pointing to a large swelling on a cow's back. He started to squeeze the lump round its base, as though it were a large boil ready to discharge. Suddenly, a creamy-yellow something, as large as my thumb, shot out and, with a sickening plop, landed on the concrete floor.

British insect life is, for the most part, reassuringly diminutive. This grub, however, was large and fascinatingly repellent, the more so because it had obviously gained its turgid obesity at the expense of the cow.

John was delighted by my look of horror. "Tha's a warble, lad" he said. And, before I had time to examine it, he'd mashed it under his boot. The mangle of stumpy legs protruding from the creamy smear made me feel quite queasy.

Such was my dramatic induction to the hidden world of parasites. But it would be a few years, in my third year at university, before I would find out more about warbles. Adult warble flies live for only a few days, during which they mate. The females then hunt out a bovine "host", and lay their eggs on hairs on its legs. Cattle seem to know that warble flies are up to no good, and when they are about they will sometimes panic and stampede. The larvae which hatch from the eggs burrow into the skin, causing quite a bit of irritation, and then migrate upwards through the connective tissues, dissolving them as they go. The Latin name for this genus of flies, *Hypoderma* derives from this under-the-skin journey. The larvae of this particular species, *Hypoderma bovis*, rest up over winter in the vicinity of the spinal canal, and feast on the epidural fat surrounding the spinal cord. In early spring they migrate to their final resting place under the skin of the back and secrete an enzyme to dissolve it. This creates a breathing hole which, as an unfortunate side effect for the farmer, greatly reduces the value of the beast's hide skin for leather. The larvae undergo a couple of moults and finally emerge as large grubs, just as John had shown me. After dropping to the ground, they pupate. A few weeks later the pupae hatch and a new fly emerges. The cycle is complete.

These days cattle warble flies are, in Western countries at least, an endangered species. They have a long period of residence within their hosts when they are susceptible to parasiticides. I have not seen another warble in all my years as a vet, which suits me fine. Once was enough. Today's organic farmers can breathe a sigh of relief that these pests were eliminated in the post-war years of over-optimistic chemical reliance. They can hitch a ride on the success of the Warble Fly Eradication Scheme. Thanks to this co-ordinated effort, cattle which could, previously, be unwitting hosts for to up to three hundred warbles each, are now warble free.

After witnessing such ghastly afflictions, I feel eternally grateful that, in cold westernised countries at least, the more dramatic human parasites have been largely eliminated. Yet were I to visit Central America or Mexico there is a chance that I could become infected by a close relative of the cattle warble fly, *Dermatobia hominis*. The larvae of this little beauty make life a misery for the people they infest, as they gnaw away at the tissues under the scalp. Those of us who endure the gloomy misery of winters in temperate latitudes would do well to ponder on the benefits they confer.

I have often wondered how Noah maintained such life forms on his amazing Ark for the benefit of later generations of mankind. Ah! You would not have me take that Ark stuff literally? Is there a middle ground? Intelligent design? Alas, the world of parasitology is replete with many gruesome torments developed by a supposedly benevolent deity bent upon intelligent design.

~

The parasites that cause the most damage to livestock are, individually, far less dramatic than warbles. Nematodes, minute worms that suck blood or chew away at the intestinal walls of sheep or cattle are, for the most part, scarcely visible to the human eye; yet they cause illness and even death because they swarm there in such vast numbers. The presence of a few is no cause for alarm, but a few thousand spell trouble. These days farmers can assess the level of threat to their grazing animals by counting the parasite eggs shed in the animals' dung. Not only is it possible to count the eggs, but also to identify which species of nematodes are present and their likely significance.

By the early '90s Otautau Vets was handling more and more dung samples brought in by farmers who saw the benefit of these faecal egg counts. Over the counter they came: in bread bags, inverted plastic gloves and even crimped baking cups. We would take these offerings into our little back-room laboratory and portion them out, soften them in a salty solution and mash them through tea strainers with a teaspoon. We could then count the nematode eggs under a microscope using a special slide with grid marks. It's amazing how much useful information can be gleaned from such unpromising material. As the lens glides over the grid it reveals a microcosm of parasite eggs, a testament to the prolificacy of internal parasites: from minute coccidian oocysts, to the bold and beautifully structured eggs of the genus *Nematodirus*. Based on our findings we could predict when it was time for the farmer to drench his animals for worms.

The eggs of some *Nematodirus* species require freezing before they will hatch. They will only emerge after the frosts of winter, not unlike the strategy of vernalization used by some plant seeds to ensure that they germinate in spring. It is an ingenious adaptation because, in temperate regions, it ensures that the larvae are triggered to hatch from their old dung patches and crawl to the succulent tips of the fresh new grass. What better launching pad to infect young lambs tucking into rich spring pastures? Reflect on these blood sucking parasites sapping the strength from those darling lambs gambolling amongst the daffodils. Before long they will suffer a black scour: blackened by their own partially digested blood as it is voided by the blood-sucking worms within them. Without treatment some will die of anaemia and dehydration. Others will fail to fatten. But can we really blame Noah for ensuring that even these little blood suckers survived the great flood? Did he really have access to freezer facilities on board the Ark to maintain his lines of *Nematodirus battus*?

It could be argued that we of Otautau Vets, facing our daily deluge of dung, were victims of our own success. Staff complained about the unsavoury stench wafting through the building. We installed an extractor fan. We insisted that the farmers wrapped their samples in clean bags before they dumped them on our front desk. But farmer laxity was not the only risk.

Vets, by the very nature of their dirty job, can become blasé about its dangers. The thoughtful bacteriologist could, with some justification, become an obsessive-compulsive hand washer and the parasitologist a food faddist. The parasitologist at the barbecue, by one definition, is the one who cuts his pork sausages longitudinally prior to cooking. *Trichinella spiralis*, a nasty parasite found in pig meat that can wreck humans, certainly justifies this caution. Vets should be fully aware of the risks from bacteria and parasites; yet for a few of them, the idle conditioning of their days in student flats overrides the sheer inconvenience of applying the principles of their new-found knowledge and the very good reasons why they, exposed to all sorts of pathogens, should have especially high standards of personal hygiene. One of our veterinary employees, a brilliant academic who subsequently left to pursue a career in research, resented being ticked off about the suspicious smears on his arms at morning tea one day. To the horror of all present he reached for the tea towel hanging by his elbow, wiped off the offending matter, and replaced it back on its rail. The ensuing chorus of protest could be politely rendered: "Hey, K~, do you realise what you've just done?"

K~ was surprisingly unabashed: "This isn't an effing girls' school, is it?"

My partners and I were on the verge of mutiny from the rest of our staff. Perhaps we had uncovered the mystery of the vanishing teaspoons. A ruling was made: henceforth any teaspoon or tea strainer disappearing from the tearoom for faecal egg counting purposes could not be returned there, no matter how thoroughly it was washed. But the next phase in the development of our faecal egg counting service rendered these mundane kitchen implements obsolete.

The process of preparing the samples was tedious. Even the glories of *Nematodirus* eggs pall on the hundredth viewing. We needed to mechanise, and Giles had some ideas. A milkshake mixer should do the job... A few days later Giles and I met at a kitchenware store in Invercargill. We found a couple of models, but they looked flimsy. "Haven't you got anything a bit more robust?" we asked. "This is going to have heavy use on a daily basis."

"We don't have any complaints from home-users about either of these models," the salesman tried to convince us, "after all, you're not going to be running them all day long, are you?"

"But it's possible we might be." Giles replied, "We'd really prefer one designed for commercial use, rather than for a home kitchen."

We turned aside to discuss our options. Sheep grazing dry summer pastures produced hard pellets of dung. We needed a machine with a lot of grunt to break these down sufficiently for the worm eggs to float out into our egg counting solution. The salesman must have overheard some of our conversation. He looked at us dubiously, glancing around to make sure no other customers were within earshot: "Hey, what sort of guys are yous?"

"Vets!" The light was dawning, but he seemed unimpressed when we disclosed the full story; alas, such a mixer was not to be had. Reluctantly, we bore our compromise purchase back to the clinic to see what we could do with it.

Overnight Giles performed one of his mechanical miracles. Our bench top ectomorph had become unrecognisable. He was now a wall-mounted warrior, complete with a hands-free lever arm and new splashguard. His blade had been modified to cut the crap. When, after several years, and thousands of shit-shakes later, the gearing started to slip, Giles modified the motor. That unpretentious little machine was still battling on ten years later—one of the best $20 investments Otautau Vets ever made.

~

A tribute to Noah: consummate stockman and supreme survivalist.

One problem with creative writing is the risk of making fundamental errors, especially when it comes to the use of humour. If you feel that by using the words "fundamental" and "creative" in a sentence relating to religious faith I am inviting trouble, you are correct.

And so, inevitably, I have been drawn—like a moth to a flame—to give a veterinary perspective on creationism. Moths are probably quite a good place to start, but since there are new species of moths being discovered practically every day, from Aotearoa to the Ruwenzori, perhaps we should gloss over Noah-the-entomologist. Besides, it's just too difficult to imagine suitable habitats aboard the Ark for porina moth, argentine stem weevil or varroa mites. The parasites, as we have seen, are very problematical. In my opinion Noah must have had a large basket hidden somewhere aboard. This would have been labelled with the Hebrew equivalent of "too hard". Let's not think about it.

I prefer to revisit my childhood picture books—the animals going in two by two. In hindsight I hadn't then appreciated Noah's consummate stockmanship. Without the use of tranquillizer darts he coaxed rhinoceri, elephants, giraffe and okapi (rediscovered by western science only last century) into the capacious hold of his magnificent Ark, plus all the parasites that in and on them dwell.

He was also, no less, an amazing traveller—prepared to go beyond the boundaries of his known world. Imagine his mighty ship ploughing through the icebergs off Tairoa Heads on his *hoiho* gathering expedition, bouncing into Botany Bay for a pair of kangaroos or lazing up the Limpopo in search of hippos; and all without the help of Pontius Pilot for those tricky estuaries. *Hoiho*, the name given by Maori to the yellow-eyed penguin, are substantial birds that he couldn't possibly have overlooked, but how Noah caught them is not recorded. What a shame that his exertions on behalf of the Dodo, the Tasmanian Thylacine and the Little Swan Island Hutia were to prove in vain.

Recent speculation by protagonists of intelligent design ingenuously explains how all this teeming life could have been crammed aboard the ark, by proposing that Noah merely required pairs of genera, not individual species: a generic "rhinoceros" rather than an Indian, White, Black, Javan or Sumatran rhino, and so on. This is precisely in agreement with my childhood picture books. Of course, this theory blithely ignores a central tenet of fundamentalists own beliefs, for surely these generics must have *evolved* (dirty word) into species later? Why not make it simpler still and take Noah's mission one further step backwards and lighten his burden to representatives of taxonomic families? This would have made for a lot more ship room. It would have been so much easier if he could have just taken his house cats and not bothered with those pesky lions and tigers. With further logic we could go to the very base of the taxonomic tree and deduce that all life as we know it descended from the basic microflora and fauna—the primordial soup—within Noah's body.

We shall never know, but perhaps we can piece it all together to our own satisfaction with a bit of education and an ounce of common sense.

I have my own theories about the parasites...

Chapter Fifteen

Holes in the Head: Windows to the Soul

Such is the human race. Often it does seem such a pity that Noah and his party did not miss the boat. – Mark Twain

One of the life forms on board Noah's Ark must have been *Coenurus cerebralis*, perhaps developing in the brain of one of his sheep. The name does not explain that *Coenurus* is the larval cyst, in sheep, of a tapeworm called *Taenia multiceps*—which infects dogs. The two names bear no resemblance because when they were named, the connection was not realised. The eggs of this tapeworm pass out in dogs' faeces and, when disintegrated and dried, they can be blown by the wind for miles. They then hatch into larvae in the intestines of sheep which have had the misfortune to ingest pasture contaminated with them. Eventually the larvae travel through the blood and take up residence in the spinal cord or, classically, the brain (hence *cerebralis*), where the cyst grows. The life cycle of the parasite is completed when another dog eats the cyst in the carcase of the sheep.

There are other tapeworm species that share similar dog-to-sheep lifecycles. *Echinococcus granulosus* is perhaps the most infamous of these. Its larval forms can develop into massive hydatid cysts in the abdominal cavity. Here they have space to grow into massive sacs containing many litres of fluid. Unfortunately, they can infect people as well as sheep and have caused many deaths and untold misery throughout history. Hydatid disease has been all but

137

eradicated in New Zealand, but only after many years of concerted effort.

It has not been recorded how Noah elected to perpetuate all these nasty tapeworms. He had several options with these multi-host parasites: via sheep infected with larval cysts, via tapeworm infested dogs or by separating the tapeworm eggs from the dog faeces and storing them. Tapeworm eggs are extremely durable and resistant to desiccation, so the latter would have been the most pragmatic solution, especially with space on board at such a premium. No matter which, humanity has no cause to celebrate the success of his efforts.

The expanding *Coenurus* cyst, by contrast, causes a variety of signs in affected sheep because the brain tissue surrounding it is slowly compressed within the bony confines of the skull. These include head tilting, walking in circles, or head pressing—where the animal presses its head hard against a wall or a post. The common name for these afflictions is "gid". If the cyst is close to the surface of the brain, the overlying bone is sometimes softened, especially in young animals.

A very valuable and strapping young Suffolk ram was brought into the Liverpool University Veterinary hospital. He was circling. What a gift for tutors trying to expand our clinical thinking!

"OK Miss Coster, if he's circling anticlockwise, which hemisphere of the brain do you expect to be affected?"...

"And if he was blind, in which eye would you expect impaired vision?"...

"How would you check a ram's eyesight? You can't exactly cover one eye and ask him to read an eye chart!" Laughter…

Later, "All right, so we think there is a space-occupying lesion somewhere in the left cranial hemisphere. What are the differentials?" At which stage gid would be mentioned along with a host of other possible causes—most of them carrying a grave prognosis.

"Well then, Mr Hardcastle, let's see if we can feel any softening of the bone." And we could!

In the end it was relatively simple surgery to make an incision in the form of an X in the skin over the softer bone, peel back the four skin flaps, break down the soft bone underneath, and remove the gelatinous cyst. The ram was much brighter the next day, perhaps relieved of a monumental headache, and over a few days he gradually gained direction and stopped circling. It was one of the more memorable moments of my clinical years at university. I particularly remembered how thrilled the farmer was when he came to collect his newly invigorated, and by now quite stroppy, ram.

There is nothing new about brain surgery. Making holes in the skulls of others is an ancient occupation. However, when the procedure is not performed by a weapon, but carefully and deliberately, presumably for curative purposes, it is described as *trephination*. Hundreds of trephined skulls belonging to Neolithic people have been found, some of which have been trephined up to six times—veritable colanders. But why did they do it? Perhaps Neolithic man suspected that the soul resided within the skull. He may not have been too far from the truth. A new science, *neurotheology* has linked electromagnetic stimulation of the temporal lobes of the brain to intense religious experiences, where 80 per cent of people become aware of a "sensed presence".

Later poets described the eyes as windows of the soul (although the idea is at least as old as Cicero), and the great Sir Isaac Newton, displaying extreme dedication to science, investigated this by inserting steel bodkins through his eyelids and calmly recording the effects. But this was mere child's play by comparison with our earlier ancestors who, by trephination, obtained far more direct access.

Closer examination has shown that these windows in Neolithic skulls were made with flint tools in one of three ways: either by patiently scraping away the bone, by cutting ever deeper in a circle, or drilling a series of small holes in a circle and then cutting the bony bridges between them.

Trephination has been performed by "primitive" tribes well into recent times, from the Pacific to the Balkans: for headaches, epilepsy, head injuries and the all-embracing category of "ritual". In 1901 the Rev. JA Crump described the technique, as practised in New Britain, where it was used to remove bone fragments and relieve the pressure of haemorrhage following trauma—reasons which would be entirely endorsed by today's top surgeons. The patients were usually casualties from inter-tribal warfare. The task was entrusted to a tribal healer or priest, using a piece of shell, shark's tooth or flake of obsidian for a trephine. The survival rate from the procedure in Melanesia was, reportedly, around seventy per cent. This compared more than favourably with the seventy-five per cent mortality achieved by St George's and Guy's hospitals in a survey of thirty-two cases between 1870 and 1877. However, without knowing the age ranges of the patients and the reasons for the operations, such comparisons can be misleading. One group comprised fit young warriors romping in a healthy, unpolluted environment; the others, most likely, were the etiolated denizens of Dickensian London.

By the middle of the twentieth century western surgeons, working in mental institutions, were opening skulls with reckless abandon—lobotomising patients with psychological disorders. Tens of thousands of these psychosurgical operations were performed in the United States alone. It was a crudely simple technique. It merely involved thrusting an ice pick between the eyeball and the eyelid, up through the bone of the orbit and directly into the frontal lobe of the brain. The instrument was then swung from side to side, effectively destroying the brain tissue. By the admission of Walter Freeman, the neurologist who invented this technique, it was "disagreeable" to watch. Nevertheless, he advised that the patients could "get up and go home within an hour or two of surgery". There might be the odd black eye as a consequence and "some minor behavior difficulties". Had Sir Isaac Newton been a little bolder in his own experiments with the bodkin, he could have lobotomised himself and changed his personality into the semblance of a passive cabbage. Victims of psychosurgery filled the psychiatric wards until the technique fell into disfavour. Besides, when tranquillizers became available in the 1950s the same effects could be produced chemically. It was far less messy.

~

Apart from the experience with the Suffolk ram, I am reminded of another instance when I needed to trephine a patient. This time it was a mare, and my trephine was rather make-shift—a hole-saw: the tool a plumber *should* use when making a hole to take a pipe through a board—but which the cruder of them don't, hoping that the dreadful crimes they commit with their hammers will remain undiscovered in the hidden corners under your sink or bath.

The mare had been dripping pus from a nostril for a long period of time. We concluded that it was most likely to be the overflow from a reservoir of pus in an infected sinus. Sinuses are bony cavities which line the skull in front of the brain and surround the nasal passages down the long muzzle of the horse. Nowadays flexible fibre-optic scopes can be passed up the nostril, enabling vets to explore the sinuses in detail and pin-point the source of such problems. However, before they were available we had to rely on cruder methods, such as tapping over the suspect sinus. Was that a healthy hollow sound, or the dull thud of a pus-filled cavity? Was there pain, or was the horse snagging back because she resented being tapped in a strange place? Such tests were often inconclusive and, if the discharge did not resolve with prolonged medical therapy, exploratory surgery, in the hope of finding the seat of the problem, was the next step.

Many horses take flight at the mere sight or smell of a vet—as readily, perhaps, as one of our Neolithic ancestors when approached by a shaman with a flint scraper. We certainly did not anticipate that our mare would stand still when we approached her with a noisy electric drill, still less when it was applied to the side of her face. So, unlike our poor ancestors, she benefited from a general anaesthetic administered by Giles. Once she was down and out, and the site of the operation shaved and prepared, I raised the skin flaps to expose the bone overlying her maxillary sinus and, carefully placing the hole-saw to avoid damaging important nerves and blood vessels, I buzzed away till I had duly removed a neat circle of bone. The ancients would sometimes keep such roundels from their own skulls on a necklace, wearing them to the grave—perhaps as an amulet—little realising that this would be a matter of enormous speculation for archaeologists a few thousand years into the future.

Through the hole I had created we could now see the outer part of the sinus cavity straddling the roots of the mare's upper molar teeth, and we flushed out the infection we expected was trapped there. It was dramatic surgery, but ultimately unsuccessful. The mare recovered well from the operation, but the discharge of pus from her nostril kept recurring. It never fully resolved. If only we'd retrieved that neat roundel of bone and placed it about her neck. That way we would not only have let out the evil spirit, but warded it off so that it couldn't jump back in again—as undoubtedly happened.

It is easy to dismiss that which we vehemently wish to avoid, and flippantly refer to "needing it like a hole in the head", but these cautionary tales should cause reflection on a misused phrase. Sometimes a hole in the head is exactly what we need.

Chapter Sixteen

Frozen Fellsides, Pregnant Distrust and Rough Justice

The Yorkshire climate is, to say the least, invigorating. True Yorkshiremen may deny this but, after becoming intimately associated with the beautiful Dales as a veterinary student, I know it to be so. It is usually office workers who tell you how much they envy your outdoor lifestyle. What greater pleasure is there than to be outdoors on a balmy summer evening and feel the caress of a warm breeze as you amble beside a lazy stretch of the Rawthey? Or wake to a bright sun on a brisk spring morning, filled with the scent of recent rain? The days when you flick along the primrose-spangled country lanes with your windows open and inhale the fresh promise of quickening hedgerows? But, in reality, those working outdoors cannot choose these moments of poesy. It is quite often at the dead of night, or in lashing rain or driving sleet, that the services of a vet are required.

There were days of drear frost when ears stung in the thin air, hands stuck to metal and feet numbed in cold rubber gumboots. Mike Harkness was TB (tuberculosis) testing wild Galloway cattle up on the fellside. I was given the exacting task of helping him to clean the brass eartags, encrusted as they were with wax and dirt, and record their numbers in a book. The restless animals plunged and reared and bellowed and banged, fighting against the pipework crush holding them. They were careless of any damage they might inflict on their own hard skulls and lashing limbs, and they imperilled our cold-befuddled fingers in the process. When we had at last finished, and the lowering sky darkened to the silent gloom of a midwinter's afternoon, and as the circulation was achingly restored to my feet thrust under the Landrover's heater, I did wonder if I was truly cut out to be a farm vet. Much of Mike's income came from the routine testing of cattle for TB or brucellosis for MAF, the Ministry of Agriculture. Indeed, most rural practices in the remoter parts of Britain relied for much of their income on this dull and, given the lack of facilities on many farms, often dangerous work. But I was starting to realise that there are few rewards without pain. If I were to enjoy the moments of pleasure from bringing a live calf into the world, I would also have to make the most of some of the worst jobs imaginable.

Although the New Zealand climate is generally milder than the British one, it is at least as wet. The very mildness permits farming to proceed without a heavy capital expenditure on winter housing for animals. This can be unfortunate for vets. Instead of calving Daisy in a cosy byre, Kiwi cow 539 is likely to be at the bottom of a paddock with only motorbike access.

It can take a while to acclimatise. Sid found the Southland winters especially trying after the heat of South Africa, and dressed accordingly. One farmer, after a visit from our newly arrived South African vet, told our receptionist that he wasn't sure which vet he'd been dealing with "because only his eyeballs were showing". The only clue was that he did have an accent. In New Zealand, New Zealanders don't have accents, so that ruled out Daryl. He could only mean Giles, Sid or me. It was amazing how farmers confused these foreign vets with their strange 'twangs'. However, in this particular instance, it could never have been Giles.

Giles had spent much of his early life as a working vet in the north of Scotland. He is, by nature, ascetic and this obliges him to eschew all creature comforts. The colder the day, the more clothes Giles casts off. By July, traditionally the coldest month in Southland, he is down to his short-sleeved shirts and ready for the start of the calving season. Mike Harkness would have been proud to accept Giles as his protégé. Disdaining the modern paraphernalia of a protective calving gown, Giles does as Mike did. He strips to the waist.

Whilst in this uncomfortable state of undress, Giles was, one winter's day, engrossed in a caesarean operation on a cow in the middle of a paddock. The slanting rain turned to sleet, and finally, snow. John, the farmer who had until then been assisting, and gallantly shielding his vet with an umbrella, had a meeting to attend. Giles had only to place the final row of skin sutures, so John left him to finish alone. Giles continued and, before leaving the farm, left a note in the milking shed with final instructions for antibiotic treatment to be picked up from the clinic. This blotchy sheet was eventually passed over the counter to Glenda, our receptionist. It was a painstaking work of spidery penmanship. It could only have been the work of either a very ancient and feeble human being, or one shivering on the verge of hypothermia. Here was hard evidence that Giles was not totally superhuman after all … but almost. Where personal hardship is concerned the rest of us had to concede that Giles was the master of stoicism and better at it than any of the rest of us.

As testosterone drains from the pages of veterinary history and women predominate in a rapidly feminising profession, heroic deeds become less valued; physical competitiveness is fading from the workplace. Daryl was never one to be outdone, but even he spurned the

146

coldness endurance challenge. I theorise that Giles runs on hot blood like penguins, whose core temperature is several degrees warmer than that of most normal human beings. Forgive my mixed metaphors, but on a winter's day, while the rest of us were rugged up, yet still as cold as frogs' tits—and not afraid to admit it—Giles sealed his lips, discarded his clothes and paraded like a penguin in summer moult. Indeed, Rosie has a picture of her husband, in swimming togs, perched on an iceberg in the glacial lake at the terminus of the Hooker Glacier at Mount Cook.

Daryl's forte was to single-handedly tackle the largest jobs in the book. A thousand deer to TB test here, 700 rams to blood test there: Daryl's your man. Indeed, he was a hard act to follow and had some loyal followers amongst our farmers. It was difficult not to disappoint one of his regulars if you happened to turn up on their farm when he was unavailable.

One of Daryl's fans owned a large sheep and beef property in the hills towards the Fiordland National Park boundary. My first visit there was to pregnancy test 500 beef cows. It promised to be, as some wag has put it: "another day at the orifice". I've already described a DY, and here was the antipodean equivalent, a dour New Zealand farmer. DNZs are a rare breed, but this DNZ was light years away from our struggling DY. His name was Hugh. Hugh ran a massive enterprise with some flair. Daryl had been extensively involved with him in an exotic beef breeding programme involving a lot of surgical embryo transfer work and numerous caesarean operations and, consequently, had developed a well-earned rapport with Hugh.

When I arrived I was immediately reminded that I was second choice: "Hello, I'm John".

147

"Hello John," (most New Zealanders say "gidday", not "hello"; unless they've attended certain upper-crust schools in Canterbury). Hugh spoke with a cultured voice, but he was obviously disappointed. "I was expecting Daryl."

"I know Hugh. I'm sorry, but I'm afraid he's away for a few days."

Hugh paused and sucked on his pipe for a bit.

"All right then, but before you start on the main mob, I'd like you to pregnancy test these."

In a side yard Hugh had a pen full of enormous Chianina heifers. Chianinas are the largest breed of cattle in the world. The average Chianina cow stands about a foot taller than a Hereford, New Zealand's commonest breed of beef cattle. But Hugh had good facilities and he organised a box for me to stand on so that I could insert my arm into the appropriate aperture. I groped around inside the first heifer for some time; Hugh seemed very concerned that these rare cattle should be pregnant. He looked the type who would, if not shoot the messenger, at least turn up the grump factor and make life unpleasant for him. Eventually I found a tiny uterus, which fell within the span of my fingers. She certainly wasn't pregnant. "Not in calf," I announced confidently. Hugh looked not best pleased. The next heifer was the same, and my pronouncement met with the same response. I was starting to feel more uncomfortable. The third one came: "I'm sorry, but she's empty [not pregnant], too." The fourth and the fifth were the same. There was a pattern here.

"OK John, they're all empty. Now that I know you can pregnancy test let's move onto the main mob."

I had my pride, "It may have been an expensive way to prove my competence". But Hugh had his reasons. He gave me a wry smile. "I'm sorry to put you

148

through it, John, but we've had young vets make mistakes before. That can be even more expensive. I had sorted those heifers out to send to the works. They're left over from our trials with exotic breeds. Unfortunately, Chianinas just aren't performing on this farm. I never even put them to the bull, so I knew they were all empty."

A few hours later I had finished the main mob. Hugh was happy with his results and I was invited in "for a bite to eat". We got on reasonably well after that.

Hugh may have been a cultured man, but that could not always be said of his staff. One of his managers was instantly recognisable as a rogue, a very personable rogue, but one surrounded by rumours of dishonesty. During his brief tenure, the cattle on the station became progressively wilder. They were restless in the yards and charged down the races at breakneck speed. Above them Roughneck hovered with a prodder connected to the electric fence unit, and he didn't hesitate to use it.

One day I turned up to pregnancy test the cows as usual. I togged up in my full-length calving gown and waterproof over-trousers and pulled on a pair of shoulder length plastic gloves. Thus accoutred, and carrying a five litre container of lubricant and a spare box of gloves, I was ready to tackle my 500 cows. No one was about, but I could hear them shifting restlessly on the other side of the shed wall. No longer were they relaxed in these yards; they were now—thanks to Roughneck and his electric wand—in a place of painful experiences. I should have been on my guard.

There was a gap between the shed wall and the race occupied by an elevated plank walk—a useful feature in any configuration of yards. In this case it also served as a stile giving access to the yard inside. As I was clambering over it, both hands full and hampered by my clinging calving gown, I heard a bellow and a crazed bull charged for the gap. In the nick of time I ducked out of line and he shot through and hurtled past my car and into the paddock beyond. Roughneck and his mates thought it was a huge joke, as I discovered when I finally caught up with them. Close calls are not entirely unexpected when you are working with beef cattle so, after a few expletives I, too, laughed it off. But I felt uneasy about this episode. What would induce an animal to act out of character like that?

It was many years later that one of the cattle hands explained what had happened. Roughneck had decided that he and his mates could have a good laugh at the expense of the vet. A particularly stroppy bull had been drafted off and provoked to distraction with the electric prodder. It was then merely a matter of timing to release him just as the vet was clambering into the yard via the only escape route for the enraged animal. Sometimes practical jokes can be taken too far. This was a case of thoughtless misjudgement rather than malicious intent; nevertheless, a hit from a 600 kg bull at full tilt could have been fatal. I have been accident prone throughout my life but, in this instance, fortune was on my side and I escaped with nothing more than depleted adrenal glands.

However, Roughneck, in his dealings with us, did not always have it his own way. One day we turned up to work to find a very sick horse in the paddock next to the clinic and a horse float [trailer] parked nearby. The horse obviously had advanced pneumonia and the prospects of it surviving were negligible. No one had made an appointment with us about seeing a very sick horse. Whose was it? Roughneck phoned later in the day. He had decided to leave his horse with us to see what we could do. He'd already tried using some antibiotics left over from a cow which died, but "they were useless" and the horse was getting worse. He didn't mind how much it cost, he wanted it treated. We wouldn't be the only vets in the world who are wary of "I don't care how much it costs". In Roughneck's case, as in so many others, the most likely reason he didn't care was because he had no intention of paying. For us there were other considerations. To leave a horse heaving its last in our paddock, right beside the main road, was inhumane and not a very good advertisement for our services. Neither would it be easy to dispose of the carcase if it died there. We persuaded Roughneck that the best option was to put it out of its misery. We would load the horse onto the float and euthanise it there. Roughneck could then come and collect the trailer and take it back to the farm to dispose of the carcase, where it would have to be buried. There is always a danger of horses euthanised with barbiturates being fed to dogs and killing them, too.

In the event Roughneck's horse died before we could inject it. A dying horse on the premises may not be a good advertisement for a veterinary practice, but a dead one is even worse. We phoned Roughneck and politely requested him to collect the carcase as soon as possible. We considered butchering it and slotting it, piece by piece, through the small apertures in the concrete lid of our offal pit. Daryl had helped me to do this to another horse once, and it wasn't the easiest or most pleasant of tasks. Besides, by this stage Roughneck was not the sort of person to whom we felt particularly obliged.

The next day the dead horse still lay in our paddock. Knowing Roughneck, if we weren't careful his float would disappear in the night, leaving the carcase for us to dispose of anyway. We had a dilemma. How do you load a dead horse onto a float? The answer proved relatively simple. We tied a long rope round the neck, passed it up the ramp, out through the side door at the front of the float and attached it to the tow bar of a four-wheel drive truck. Unfortunately, we were unable to fold the legs and they remained rigidly extended in rigor mortis. As the truck inched forwards and the body slowly ascended the ramp, we had to rotate it. It came to rest with its back on the floor of the trailer and its legs in the air.

It took a few more phone calls before Roughneck condescended to collect his loaded float. A whiff was beginning to blow about our premises. Had Roughneck had the last laugh? Then, one morning, the float had vanished. I often wonder what the occupants of any vehicles following it on its journey home would have thought. Instead of the familiar sight of a horse's buttocks and tail swaying above the tailgate, a pair of hoofs projected skywards. An upside-down horse? What on earth was going on?

Chapter Seventeen

Death and Dignity

Life is pleasant. Death is peaceful. It's the transition that's troublesome. – Isaac Asimov

Roughneck's horse met an undignified end. At such times, it seems as though a vet's life disproportionately revolves around being a handmaiden to death or, worse still, a harbinger of death. If your cover as a vet is blown at some social function, one of the commoner responses you will elicit from an empathetic member of the public is "I could never be a vet; you have to put animals to sleep". A more direct person will dispense with the euphemism. "I don't know how you vets can kill animals." I have to remind myself that, by frequent exposure, it is possible to become inured to death.

As a child, I could disregard death. It never touched me personally in my small nuclear family. When things died they became flat. I was convinced of this, the evidence was before my eyes every time I crossed the busy streets of Liverpool. The dead sparrows were flat; the dead pigeons were flat; the dead cats were flat. If I had been brought up in the country, I would no doubt have had some other equally misleading misconception.

The spiritual dimension to death was brought home to me when I was a bit older.

Within the four brick walls of our back garden it was safe to use an air rifle. My brother and I shot at targets and empty tin cans suspended on string. We chewed up wads of paper into papier-mâché pellets, a humane but time-consuming method of eliminating blue bottles. But the hunter is alive in most boys and one day, seeing a pigeon alight on the gutter three stories above my head I watched as it strutted and peered over the edge. My air rifle was loaded. I drew a bead on the jerking neck silhouetted against the bright sky and squeezed the trigger. It was a spontaneous shot at a moving target and I hit it! The pigeon pitched forward and spiralled down right beside me. It was only a fleeting moment of exhilaration. As I cradled the warm, limp body I saw the life drain from its blood-red eye, and I felt a deep sadness about what I had done. I had killed gratuitously.

I still have reservations about blood sports and rip and yank fishing orgies. The boundaries between killing to eat, killing to eradicate pests and preserve the environment, and killing for fun, are sometimes blurred. Euthanasia confronts vets daily, and is distinctly different.

Euthanasia should be a dignified act of mercy. It may appear callous to say it, but I have felt absolutely right injecting an overdose of barbiturate into the vein of an old, arthritic Labrador or a paraplegic road accident victim. I am relieving suffering. It is more distressing if the animal is healthy, young and friendly and the procedure is being performed as a matter of convenience for the owner, but then, like most vets, we usually tried to find a home for it. Occasionally this was not possible, but at least the final process was humane. Better the owner who has faced up to their responsibilities in this way than dumped their pet somewhere in the wild in the hope that it will survive— often a cruel recipe for a slow death by starvation.

In most cases euthanasia involves giving a lethal injection into the cephalic vein on the forearm of the dog or cat. It may sound simple, but it is one of the more demanding duties a vet has to perform. Finding the vein to inject an anaesthetic whilst under the bright lights of the clinic with an experienced animal nurse holding the animal, is one thing; but sometimes it is either less stressful for the pet, or the owner's choice, to have the vet call in and do the deed at home. As the vet concerned, you are usually very much on your own. It's a matter of staff resources: the practice can't spare the nurse to help you out when she is required at the clinic to assist with all the other ops lined up.

When you finally reach your destination, you may find all sorts of obstacles to a pleasant outcome: the dog has cardiac failure and his veins are collapsed; he can't move far, but he's not going to take that prick in his leg lying down; the old lady can't hold him; no, the coal cellar is his favourite place and there is no other lighting apart from this failing torch. If it's a cat: he's just this moment disappeared; he seems to know what's going on and we can't get him out from under this very low super king-sized bed; he's just scratched my arm, see if you can catch him etcetera, etcetera. You are expected to cope, as in: "Well, you're the vet. That's why I called you."

~

Every vet will have a disaster story concerning euthanasia. One of my first memories relates to my days as a student filling in the summer holidays for the obligatory number of weeks of "seeing practice" before qualifying. I was commandeered by Mick, one of the young Watford vets, to help him put down a Pyrenean Mountain Dog which had bitten a neighbour. In England in the early 1970s these dogs were the latest fashion accessory for those who liked big dogs or wanted something large and white to lie on their shag-pile carpet.

While PMDs may be ideal for bounding round the mountains and protecting flocks of sheep from wolves and bears, they are not exactly suited to life in a bed-sit. The monotony of such an existence and lack of exercise tends to make them grumpier than usual. This, combined with their massive size and guarding instincts, can present a formidable challenge to any visitor, let alone one smelling of vet.

As a student I revelled in seeing how such jobs were handled. Seeing practice with an experienced vet was all fun and no responsibility. The current PC world of academia would rather students confined their extramural experience to model practices, preferably those handling referrals in a strictly approved, evidence based, scientific manner. It has always been my contention that we learn best from our mistakes, and nearly as well from other people's—so the best learning opportunities often arise from the least likely sources.

The block of flats certainly looked unpromising territory for a PMD. Mick and I pounded up the echoing stairwell trying not to inhale too deeply. The whole area had been liberally claimed by tom cats and they had been spraying within on an industrial scale. Ah, that ammoniacal reek and the brown dingy linoleum bring back memories; who could possibly choose to spend their life in small animal practice in the deprived areas of a big city?

A fat and, yes, distinctly grouchy Pyrenean Mountain Dog weighing over 50 kg guarded the top of the final narrow flight of stairs that we ascended, by necessity, in single file—right to the top garret. Mick led the way, confidently at first. I felt safe behind him. He was, after all, a strapping, young, rugby-playing vet;

but he faltered as we came to the top. He had mistakenly assumed that PMD would be under the control of his owner. Unfortunately, the latter fell into the seven stone weakling category. He had probably purchased PMD in the hope that people would stop kicking sand in his face. I'm sure they did for a while; but it was obvious that our hero had become terrified of his own dog and could do nothing to restrain him.

By the lights of Sir Walter Scott we were now confronted by a very *wrathful* dog. Charles Atlas himself would have stepped back and beaten a dignified retreat; and so did we. A full frontal, bare-handed assault was not on. We considered our options. PMD was aroused and suspicious and, under these circumstances, seven-stone weakling informed us there was no way he would take food laced with drugs. Besides, the whole process would take hours.

You can't expect an England Rugby Union trialist to admit defeat in the face of such an overt challenge. M's dander was up. He managed to convey to seven stone weakling that we would be back with a dog-catcher. In essence this is a long pole with a noose on the end. The idea is to slip the noose over the dog's head and pull it tight. If you are strong enough you can keep the dog secure at pole's length and unable to reach you. There are, however, a couple of drawbacks with dog catchers. One is that no dog enjoys a tight noose around its neck. Aggressive dogs become more aggressive and PMD was no exception. Once committed, you must have the strength and determination to win. The other drawback is that both your hands are fully occupied, so you need an assistant. The assistant needs to be able to reach the dog and on the narrow stairway this was not easy. Even super fit Mick was struggling to push PMD upstairs on the pole.

PMD was choking, his tongue was going blue and he was more than ever determined to kill us. The blank eyes of a dog in kill mode are truly terrifying. He fought against the pole like a great shark threshing on the end of a gaff. He voided his bowels and bladder. Their contents were kicked and splashed onto us as we struggled beneath him. Barbiturates have to be injected into a vein, but finding the vein in such circumstances is impossible.

We had anticipated this and planned accordingly. It was now my job to inject a morphine-based horse anaesthetic into any part of PMD's musculature. I had to be supremely careful that I wouldn't be knocked or in some other way accidentally discharge the injection into one of us. At last I found a piece of leg and carefully thrust the needle through a felted mat of ungroomed hair and into the muscle beneath. Keeping his distance, Mick carefully released PMD from the noose. Within minutes he relaxed and Mick was finally able to inject a lethal dose of barbiturate directly into his heart. He was dead in an instant.

We were now faced with the nightmare of wrestling PMD into a polythene body bag and carrying him down the stairs and past the stares of the tenants in the lower flats. They had been summoned by the thumping melee above them but, habituated by a thousand gangster movies and perhaps (who knows?) similar comings and goings up and down those stairs, they seemed unmoved by the sight of two spattered, shabby men descending from on high bearing a full body bag.

A dead weight is an awkward burden, and the dénouement was inevitable. Before their very eyes, the black polythene split, and a soiled, furry carcase cascaded onto the cat-pee landing. For some time Mick and I had been controlling ourselves and upholding, with some difficulty, the solemn standards of professionalism expected on such occasions. But, we had escaped from a surreal situation of some danger and our sense of relief eventually broke out in a very unprofessional outburst of hysterical laughter. We laughed so much that we came close to adding our own contributions to the urine drenched linoleum. That would have been triple whammy for our spectators, but they seemed to understand. One of them muttered: "Thank goodness someone's at last done something about that bastard." There seemed to be a general consensus about that.

~

As in so many other veterinary endeavours, the unpromising task of euthanasia can bring unexpected rewards.

It was the end of a long day, but our receptionist, Karen, volunteered to accompany me and lend a hand. Cassie, an old and much-loved bearded collie had had a stroke. She was fully conscious but unable to walk. I had never met her before, but I knew that she was very special; indeed she had been a New Zealand champion. Her tail flapped weakly on the floor as I greeted her.

The moment I clipped the hair off her leg I knew that I was in trouble. Cassie's circulation was poor and the vein I would have to use was not visible. In circumstances like this it is sometimes a matter of experience to guess where exactly the vein lies; but alas, luck was not with me that day. I tried the other leg, irrelevantly wondering which part of my autonomic nervous system was responsible for the large beads of sweat running down my furrowed brow and blurring the inside of my glasses. I have had people poking around trying to find my own veins and I didn't want to put Cassie or her owner through too much of that. So far I had only succeeded in getting enough barbiturate into her circulation to make her drowsy. She lay peacefully as her owner stroked her.

Fortunately there are alternatives, and I carefully slipped some of the solution into her liver. A routine euthanasia, which should have taken a few seconds, was now going to take half an hour. In fact over an hour passed before Cassie took her last breath and drifted away, across the rainbow bridge her owner talked about.

During this time Cassie's owner, initially distraught and thinking that I had, as she later put it, "stuffed up", gradually adjusted to her loss. By the end of an hour the three of us had debated our beliefs, agreed to differ, and solved many of the world's problems. Cassie's prolonged but serene departure had brought us together.

Financially it was an unrewarding exercise for all concerned. Time is costly. None of us has much to spare these days. However, sometimes benefits cannot be quantified financially. Opportunities for personal growth arise unexpectedly. We need to recognise them for what they are, and not resent the time they take when they come our way.

~

One of our loyal and favourite farming clients seemed to live their home life surrounded by pet dogs. James' and Sue's living area was a clutter of expensive but battered leather furniture, tumbled books, and the homely warmth of an Aga cooker. Though theirs was a solidly Southland family, they could have stepped out of *Country Life* magazine. Quite often, after a long job in their sheep yards, I was invited in for a cup of tea and, inevitably and irresistibly, I enjoyed some of Sue's choice home baking—followed, undesirably, by middle age spread. Finding a seat among the cushions, magazines and other assorted papers could be a problem. Humphrey lazily reclined on "his" couch and, unless sternly reprimanded by Sue, his mistress, he refused to move out of the way, although his tail usually thumped the leather in welcome.

Humphrey was a much favoured Labrador, but over the years he had slowed down and one day Sue warned me that his time was drawing near and please could I be ready to come and give him a dignified send off? Duly, that day came. The family gathered round, and Humphrey hardly stirred as he departed this world. After her final, farewell stroke of his soft ears, Sue brushed aside her tears and asked me if I'd care to join the family for a cup of tea. Invariably, on other euthanasia missions, I had refused such requests, and so I declined, saying that I thought it would be better for me to leave her and the family with Humphrey to get over their grief. Sue, however, was insistent, "Please John, we'd love you to stay."

"But what about Humphrey?"

She looked over to Humphrey's peaceful hulk. "Oh, he'll be alright. Humphrey can lie in state while we have our tea!"

Sharing that cup of tea with Humphrey's caring and humane owners was a rare privilege. If only we all had such a balanced attitude to life and death.

Chapter 18

Prussic Acid, Polecats, Possums and Tits

These days vets are required to be very circumspect about the powerful drugs at their disposal. Things were far more relaxed not so long ago. In my university days it was entertaining for veterinary students, returning from the long vacation breaks, to trade stories about the more dramatic moments they had experienced while seeing practice with different vets in various parts of Britain.

Richard, my friend from South Wales, recounted the unbelievable technique used by a very old and backward veterinarian for the destruction of aggressive cats. Admittedly, it is very difficult to restrain a cat in a demonic rage. Cat bites and scratches are painful and notoriously prone to infection. Finding small veins on a moving target can be an interesting challenge, even with the inventive use of towels and jacket sleeves for restraint. Often it is more humane to inject the cat directly into its heart or a kidney than persisting, as a matter of professional pride, in trying to find an elusive vein. These larger organs are easier targets, and also result in near instantaneous death, far better than vain vein attempts... but, in reality, such efforts may not be appreciated by nervous cats, nor the staff who have to try and avoid being bitten and scratched while trying to restrain them.

Richard's vet used Prussic acid. As the caged cat spat and snarled at him he squirted this lethal compound into its mouth, causing rapid death from cyanide poisoning. The danger to himself or his staff was appreciable. Prussic acid was one of the Nazi's favourite chemicals for mass murder. Where on earth had Richard's vet obtained it?

Strange as it may seem, tight control over nasty chemicals is a relatively recent phenomenon. In Chaucer's day (late fourteenth century) it was easy to obtain poison from an apothecary. In *The Pardoner's Tale* one of the felons used the pretext of needing it to kill the rats and a polecat that he claimed were killing his hens. It all ended in mass murder.

Control of drugs is much stricter these days and, despite occasional requests from members of the public, vets are not legally permitted to hand out powerful drugs like barbiturates for general use. If you, like the felon in Chaucer's tale, want to "quell" your rats, or poison the polecat eating your chooks, don't expect your vet to supply you with "strong and violent" poisons. And if you have a vicious dog you want out of the way, we cannot legally supply you something to "slip into his food", because how are we to know you're not going to slip it into a bottle of Pinot for your wife and her new boyfriend? Human nature doesn't change.

~

Polecats have a powerful hold on our cultural memory. Their depredations on poultry were not confined to the pages of Chaucer; they have been persecuted throughout history. In some parishes, rewards were offered for their destruction. The expression "stink like a polecat" was widely used in my childhood yet polecats had, by then, become extremely rare in the wild and were restricted to isolated corners of Wales. However, in a domesticated form they live on as ferrets—still used for rabbiting, and as pets. The fitch varieties, selected for their beautiful pelts, were farmed quite extensively in New Zealand in the 1980s as farmers desperately sought ways to generate income while the sheep industry slumped. Several barns and sheds around Western Southland were set up with fitch cages. Vets quickly learned to anticipate their lightening reactions and avoid their needle-sharp teeth when they were presented for vaccinations (they are particularly prone to canine distemper) or with various ailments. The polecat stench became quite familiar to us. One local veterinary practice even specialised in de-sexing fitches and surgically removing the anal glands responsible for their quite overpowering scent. Thus prepared, they were exported to Asia as pets. Lithe, lively and intelligent: the very qualities that make them such lethal hunters in forest and field, suited them well to the confined human warrens of Singapore.

In the wild, polecats, ferrets and escaped fitches, like their cousins—stoats and weasels—kill indiscriminately and gratuitously. After the early settlers introduced rabbits to New Zealand they multiplied to such an extent that they threatened pastoral industries. The introduction of stoats and weasels to control rabbits was, in turn, equally ill-advised. For stoats and their allies New Zealand's unique ground-nesting birds, such as kiwi, weka, kakapo and takahe, were easier pickings than rabbits. And, since these vicious predators are capable climbers, even tree-nesting birds, which evolved without effective defence strategies against them, have suffered alarmingly as their nests have been plundered by them and other introduced pests like rats, possums and feral cats.

Sadly, the bush, once reverberant with birdsong, is now largely silent; yet in the nineteenth century

164

teachers in Wellington complained that they had to close the school windows to exclude the noisy birds, so their pupils could hear them.

I can sympathise with Sid who emigrated from a country romping with spectacular wildlife to New Zealand, where we carefully foster the twilight remnants of an ornithologically spectacular fauna in the hope that more effective pest management strategies will be developed for the future. "New Zealand is a beautiful country, John, with chocolate-box scenery. But when you open the lid you find that there never were many chocolates and that most of them have already been eaten."

Ferrets and possums are vectors for bovine tuberculosis, so it is fortunate that the interests of conservationists and farmers coincide. Few New Zealanders do not want them eliminated. Should modern technology give us the means, it is to be hoped that we can look forward to the restoration of our glorious dawn chorus and, for the best of reasons, that the voices of our teachers will be drowned out once more.

~

New Zealand in its unspoilt state, before the arrival of man, could lay claim to some spectacular and unique bird life, but the number of taxa represented were rather limited when compared to those seen on the larger continental land masses. Sid's chocolate-box metaphor can be elaborated by focusing on just one family of birds.

New Zealand suffers from an extreme dearth of tits. Even the perky little New Zealand tomtit (*Petroica macrocephala*) is not a proper tit. England has a far superior array of tits: enough to make a fanatical twitcher drool. Go on, let me boast about them Sid! We've heard enough about all those boring old baboons, giraffes, elephants and lions. Let me tell you about British tits …

In my childhood our garden, deep in the smoky heart of Liverpool, was graced with winter visits from those shameless little blue tits (*Parus caerulus*) which pierced the foil caps of milk bottles and tapped off the cream. Great tits (*Parus major*) and coal tits (*Parus ater*) acrobatically pecked at the strings of peanuts my mother hung for them, well clear of the coggers' moggies which, nevertheless, prowled optimistically beneath. Away from the cities, marsh and willow tits flit in forests, bearded tits frolic in the fens and long-tailed tits shyly build feather-lined retreats in thorny thickets. Amongst the pines of the Rothiemurcus Forest in Scotland, the true tit voyeur might even ogle a perky little crested tit (*Parus cristatus*) prying seeds from cones or, as had been my luck, chance upon a lively pair disporting on a well stocked bird table. Sadly, it would only befall the luckiest of twitchers to glimpse a penduline tit. They don't hang out in Britain that often (there being only the one record, from 1966).

Chapter Nineteen

Mutation or Mutilation

Veterinarians should not perform surgical procedures for purely cosmetic purposes. Where animals carry inherited defects that compromise their welfare or that of their prospective progeny, veterinarians are expected to give sound genetic counselling and management advice in the best interests of the animal and its progeny. Veterinary Council of New Zealand Handbook 2006.

In mediaeval times royalty were entertained by court jesters. These were physically deformed, dwarfed, or insane people sold into the homes of the nobility by poor families who could not afford their upkeep. They were regarded as property to be on-sold, disposed of, or inherited at the whim of their owners. An ability to clown, do acrobatics, contort or versify enhanced their value. Cardinal Wolsey's "Patch" was worth a thousand pounds when he was donated to King Henry VIII.

Long after this fashion declined, Victorians were titillated by fair-ground freak shows and entertained by visits to "lunatic" asylums like Bedlam.

This predilection lives on in our fondness for bizarrely deformed pets: the sleek lines of wild fish degraded into the grotesque pop-eyed deformities favoured by some aquarists; the free-bounding, natural athleticism that should be the natural inheritance of any dog, spurned for that crippled, wheezing freak. Ridiculous breed standards ensure the genetic degradations become ever more extreme: shorter legs, longer backs, compressed noses, and so on.

Pathological mutations that would spell disaster for any wild animal are eagerly selected for their novelty value.

One example would be the Shar-Pei breed, familiar to many TV viewers as the wrinkly star on toilet tissue adverts. A website promoting the breed warns: *unless you are ready to commit the time and necessary finances for potential medical problems, a Shar-Pei may not be for you.* Such breeds would seem to be a vet's dream, but in reality most vets I know despair of treating the chronic skin, skeletal and other problems associated with these and other canine monstrosities. There will always be some, unfortunately, who embrace the opportunities created by this escalating freak market.

Miss Joshua, my demanding final year tutor at university, had firm views about the ethics she expected of the vets she trained—especially those who might be drawn into the shadowy world of dog breeding. She knew what she was talking about, because she was a dog breeder herself. We were instructed to firmly advise any clients who presented puppies with genetic defects to neuter the parents and offspring to prevent further dissemination of the faulty genes.

Hers was the perspective of a generation later condemned as arrogant. How people resent that "I know best" attitude of the old-style professionals, be they doctors or vets. Their advice may have been sound, but the pendulum has swung—perhaps too far the other way. These days the business ethos prevails. "Keeping your clients happy" is much the easier and more profitable path to tread when your client, the dog or cat breeder, is solely motivated by short-term gain. By these lights, it would be poor business to suppress the breeding that creates some of the more than 30,000 genetic defects that have now been identified in pedigree dogs. No wonder there is a burgeoning demand for pet vets. Astute business-minded practice owners (increasingly, these days, not veterinarians) no doubt clap their hands with glee at the prospect of multiple plastic surgery corrections with each litter of Shar-Peis that land on their examination room tables.

I deplore this exploitation. The Kennel Clubs in Britain and America have, with their ridiculous breed standards, moved the basis for selection from function to fashion. Dachshunds bred for longer backs and shorter legs have increasing spinal problems. Bulldogs bred for massive heads require caesarean births. German Shepherds bred for sloping haunches are prone to hip dysplasia. Pedigree is as poor a measure of worth, if not value, in the canine world as it is in the human. If you don't know the breeder and the nature of the dogs they breed, my advice—and I can hear a lot of tut-tutting here—is give a home to a mongrel.

One way to short-cut the genetic pathway to deformity is to create it surgically. Some mediaeval court jesters were manufactured in this way: break a limb or two and set them at an amusing angle. Foot binding persisted in China till relatively recently. More random disfigurement can still be had in Germany: *Mensur* is a form of controlled duelling with knives designed to inflict "honourable" facial scars. We once looked with incredulity at primitive tribes with their lip plates and stretched ear lobes, but we now indulge ourselves in fashionable body piercing, and pasty-faced young men parade our streets with ear inserts with the dimensions of serviette rings. For adults, in a society of breast implants and Prince Alberts, this is very much a matter of free choice. For our children and animals it is different.

In some countries it is still legal to crop the ears of dogs—especially favoured for Dobermanns and Great Danes—to make them look more vicious. This is not a minor surgical procedure; it involves removing a large portion of the ear flap, naturally hanging in these breeds, so that the remaining portion sticks up. A full anaesthetic is required. Vets in America used to do this operation routinely; however, it is regarded as unethical for vets in New Zealand and Britain to perform unnecessary surgical mutilations. According to the professional codes of conduct of most western jurisdictions it should not be permissible, but such matters are always open to legal interpretation.

~

Unwittingly, I once perpetrated an act of mutilation on an English Bull Terrier. The owner, a tough looking Yorkshire coal miner, brought Herman in with an aural haematoma. It is a common condition; rugby forwards sport untreated aural haematomas as a badge of honour. Herman's ear flap was full of blood. He looked miserable and shook his head violently. Rugby forwards have such thick necks that this is not possible. Besides, they disdain pain and like their ears to scar and pucker into disfiguring cauliflower growths—battle scars—best displayed under a shaved scalp: a form of *Mensur* in all reality.

For dogs with aural haematomas the usual veterinary procedure was to drain the blood under a general anaesthetic and place numerous cross-stitches through the full thickness of the flap to prevent it filling again. In dogs, the initiating cause is usually an ear infection rather than another forward's skull. The infection causes the head shaking which, in turn, causes a blood vessel in the ear flap to rupture and so to a vicious spiral of more head shaking. It is, therefore, very important to check for and treat any underlying ear infection, as well as to tackle the obvious haematoma.

Craig, my boss at the time, was keen to try a new technique, which involved placing stiff card on each side of the flap and stapling through the whole lot. It was certainly quicker to do, and seemed to have been well tolerated by Herman. But when it came to removing the card and staples ten days later, I was alarmed to see the end of Herman's ear slough off as I pulled away the card supports—right under the gaze of his craggy owner. The circulation to the tip of the ear flap had obviously been compromised. Fortunately, apart from the missing bite-sized chunk, it had healed well. Expecting Mr Miner to be distressed, even angered, by his dog's now less than perfect appearance, I was amazed to hear an "Eee 'erman, tha' looks a reet champion." He was thrilled by Herman's new, rugged look. How unpredictable people are.

We reverted to the old cross-stitching after that, bearing in mind that someone like Mrs Farback might not be quite as forgiving if the same fate befell Chintzywig, her miniature poodle.

~

Recently, there has been a longstanding debate about that commonest of mutilations: tail docking of pups. What an enormous amount of drivel has been written and spoken about the merits or otherwise of this procedure. I can find no rationale for the proponents' position beyond an innate desire to meddle with nature. Their strongest argument boils down to eliminating the risk of working dogs injuring their tails. It has never

171

been the normal practice to dock the tails of sheep dogs, and I worked for over thirty years in a district where thousands of them daily mustered the rough hill blocks and jump endlessly in and out of sheep and cattle yards. Other injuries were common, but tail injuries in working dogs are rare. They are seen far more commonly in pet dogs, usually as the result of getting them jammed in doors.

Why remove tails? In the course of our lives we commonly cut our fingers, but no one suggests that amputation is the best way to avoid this. Tails are useful. Watch the tail of a dog turning at speed, and the way it is used for balance. Besides, a wagging tail is a joy to behold.

One day I managed to persuade the owner of a Fox Terrier not to dock the tails of a litter of pups. I was aware that I was in danger of getting into the "I know best" trap, but we had a complete wee foxy of our own, so I really felt I did. A few years later he reminded me of this when he brought his dog in for vaccination: "Best rabbiter I've ever bred." he commented. "Do you remember you persuaded me not to dock his tail?" I couldn't, but I wondered what was coming next. "I'm so glad we didn't; now I can follow his tail through the long grass. With my other dog I never know where he is!"

Gradually the dog tail dockers have lost ground, and tail docking is now totally illegal in Scotland, only legal for "working dog breeds" in England and Wales (what a cop-out!), and "an unnecessary surgical alteration with subsequent animal welfare compromise" in New Zealand. Who said the Scots were a barbarous race?

But where do we draw the line? Fundamentalist animal rights activists are now calling to ban the tail

172

docking of lambs. This procedure is carried out when lambs are 2 – 6 weeks old. The tails of undocked sheep, when they are grazing lush pastures, readily become contaminated with faeces and are a choice target for blowflies. Meat eating maggots emerge from the eggs they lay and cause severe suffering and even death. There are few more revolting sights than a seething mass of stinking maggots writhing in a wound. The temporary suffering caused by tail docking lambs is manifestly preferable to a slow and agonising death from flystrike. The balance between welfare, convenience and tradition when considering mutilations to farm animals is, these days, under constant review. Mulesing of sheep, tail docking of cows, debeaking of poultry, teeth clipping of pigs and castration in most farmed species: all have been put under the magnifying glass.

While these debates continue, the biggest irony for me is our unquestioning acceptance of circumcision for male human infants. This, if done for non-medical reasons, should be entirely unacceptable on rational and ethical grounds. Isn't it strange that babies, supposedly made in the image of the perfect God worshipped by their parents, should require surgical improvement? And yet this mutilation is an unchallenged tenet of some religions and cultures.

Although there has been a great deal written about the unacceptability of female circumcision in western societies, I can't see OECD politicos leaping in to legislate the cause of helpless male infants subjected to this painful and pointless mutilation. Male circumcision is a taboo subject; and, I would venture to suggest, it is rather more important than tail docking of puppies.

The debates will continue. Unfortunately, the only ones who cannot join either of these discussions are those most affected by them.

Chapter Twenty

Killing Fields and Swingletrees

All interest in disease and death is only another expression of interest in life. – Thomas Mann

I was digesting my dinner one summer's evening when the phone rang: "Hi, are you the duty vet?" to which I reluctantly, but professionally, yielded my reply:

"Yes, carry on."

"Can you come quickly? My heifers are going down like flies." It was the phone call vets dread.

"Who am I talking to?"

"It's Dave, at Waicola. Remember? You were here a couple of days ago putting old 97's hip back in."

"Just bear with me a moment Dave, I need to get an idea of what's going on in case I need to pick up anything special from the clinic. Are they dying?"

"A couple have, but some are just sitting and there are a few looking sick."

My mind raced. They would be on grass, not crop, at this time of year. It was unlikely to be nitrate poisoning, one of the commonest reasons for sudden deaths. "Have they recently been moved onto a new paddock?"

"I moved them into a fresh paddock near the shed this morning."

"Are there any other symptoms Dave? Are they thrashing around, or excitable at all? Are they scouring?"

"No, they just sit down and die."

It had to be something they'd eaten. I couldn't think past nitrate poisoning, although we rarely saw it, but it was possibility if, say, a paddock of lush grass by

175

the shed had been overloaded with effluent. I wouldn't know till I got there.

"All right Dave, I'll be there in about half an hour, I'll have to pick up some extra drugs from the clinic on the way through. If you can move the healthy ones into another paddock while you're waiting it might be a good idea." It would also give him something to do. Half an hour is a long time to wait while your valuable animals die around you.

I dusted off a bottle of Methylene Blue crystals. It had sat on our shelves for years. We held it in stock "just in case" we had an outbreak of nitrate poisoning. This messy dye can be dissolved in water and injected straight into the jugular vein. It neutralises the nitrites circulating in the blood of animals that have eaten too much nitrate-rich food. Nitrites smother haemoglobin, robbing blood of its ability to carry oxygen. In effect, cattle stricken by nitrate poisoning die of chemical asphyxiation. At first they breathe more rapidly to compensate but, when 80% or more of their haemoglobin has been converted to useless met-haemoglobin, they die.

I played this over in my mind as I drove to Dave's farm and thought of the other symptoms I could expect to see. When haemoglobin is converted into met-haemoglobin, the blood loses its bright red colour and becomes a chocolate brown. Chocolate brown blood would clinch the diagnosis. I had only read about this; all the suspected nitrate poisonings I had previously encountered had been dead before I arrived on the scene, and the chocolate colour fades after death. But nothing is ever as clear-cut as textbook descriptions. I anticipated there would be the usual variability of symptoms that go with any poisoning—depending how much was ingested, how rapidly and how long ago—

questions to which the answers are seldom known. There might be gasping and rapid breathing. There might also be muscle tremor, weakness, staggering, a weak pulse and terminal convulsions. And then again, there might not.

When I arrived at the farm, there were none of these signs. Dave was reasonably calm. A calm owner always makes it easier for a vet to focus on the job in hand. He had revised his losses. He thought there were now four or five dead. I noted a similar number sitting down in their clean paddock of lush grass. There were no poisonous plants I could hang a diagnosis on, however Dave told me that he'd just discovered that the heifers had broken into his fertilizer shed and got into some bags of urea.

Could that be the problem?

Yes, it most certainly could. Although urea is frequently added to poor quality feedstuffs for cattle, it has to be extremely well mixed in so that each animal ingests no more than a few grams. For animals not accustomed to it, even small amounts are fatal. I'd had absolutely no experience of urea poisoning, but I knew someone who had and I fervently hoped he would be on the end of the line when I rang. Fortune favoured me:

"Sid, I suspect I've got a mass outbreak of urea poisoning at Dave's place. We have a few dead and sick. Any ideas?" I could almost hear his mind whirring over the line, and then, after a long pause:

"…That's not good John, we must try and get vinegar into them. The urea breaks down into ammonia in the gut… vinegar will help to neutralise it. I'll see how much I can get from the supermarket and come and give you a hand. You could try your Methylene Blue, just in case. Nitrate poisoning could look similar, but given the history it's almost certainly the urea.

Methylene Blue won't do any harm, but I don't think it will do much good."

He was right about that. By the time he arrived I looked like a woad-dyed ancient Briton. The Methylene Blue stained everything in sight, but it had made no difference to the cows I had treated. There were six dead now, and about the same number down. Dave had brought a bottle of vinegar from the house, and rung round his neighbours, and they were now turning up in the late evening light to give a hand with what vinegar they had gleaned from their cupboards. Sid had cleaned out Otautau's supermarket. "It looks a bit hopeless, John. We need at least ten bottles per animal." With all the vinegar in the district we only had sufficient to treat one-and-a-half heifers. "Never mind, thanks for coming along anyway." There were quite a few spectators by now and I really appreciated Sid turning up to share my ignominy.

We set to and passed a stomach-tube (smooth transparent tubing about the diameter of standard household hosepipe) up the nostril of one of the last sick-looking heifers sitting in front of us. When we were sure it was in the right place and not entering her lungs, we tipped our bottles of vinegar into her.

This is a story without a happy ending. The one and a half heifers we were able to treat both died. In the words of my trusty copy of *Blood and Henderson's Veterinary Medicine*: "Treatment is unlikely to be effective but the oral administration of a weak acid such as vinegar may reduce the amount of ammonia absorbed." Sometimes, as a vet, you are on a hiding to nothing. And then the self-questioning begins.

I wish it hadn't been on Dave's farm. He and his wife had experienced a string of bad luck since they'd moved there the previous autumn. Nothing that Sid or I had done had made any difference. The final toll was ten heifers dead, and there was the distinct possibility that those that recovered would abort their calves. The only consolation was that it could have been worse. Dave had been philosophical throughout, in the best farming tradition. But understanding the financial pressures some of these young entrepreneurial dairy families were under puts greater pressure on the vet to achieve a good result. I had done all I could, but it wasn't good enough.

A few days after this incident, I was introduced, at a school social, to an English immigrant who had settled on a dairy farm near Dunedin.

"You might like to meet John, Ray. John's a vet from Southland."

Like most vets I prefer not to talk shop and try to avoid veterinary topics at social events. However, the hostess had done her part and started the ball rolling. It was one that Ray soon stopped.

"I don't use a vet. I do all my own vetting."

Short of telling him or her that they are a waste of space, it is the one of the best put down lines to use on a vet. That was, more or less, the end of the conversation.

I privately seethed later. What would Ray have done if his heifers started to go down like flies? Given my recent efforts he would have saved himself quite a lot of money by not calling a vet. On the other hand, by involving his vets, Dave had a good understanding of exactly what had happened, the long-term risks and perhaps some peace of mind as a result. He could also have filed a plausible insurance claim.

Most vets are proud of their profession, but that is very different from being arrogant. Too many times we end up in hopeless situations, as I did on Dave's farm, which serve to remind us of our fallibility, something I

179

would never deny. Ray, an arrogant man, was perhaps guilty of judging me by his own standards.

Even the best of us cannot cure everything. The best we can do is get the message out to others so that these preventable accidents are avoided. Effective communication with his clients is one of the key responsibilities of any rural veterinarian.

~

I have fond memories of my early years in Otautau. They were relatively relaxed until the sheep farming recession of the 1980s and the dairy farming revival of the 1990s combined to change the face of Southland farming forever. But there were always those moments: Jim Turnbull had a "couple" of beef cows down and would I call in to have a look?

It turned out to be an interesting "look", and I've kept the case notes to this day…

It was a glorious February afternoon in 1980 when I drove to Jim's farm. It was set on the flats between the Takitimu mountains, and the Fiordland hills across the other side of the Waiau river.

High summer: the sweet smell of cut grass wafted through my windows. I breezed past patchwork paddocks: tawny, sage and verdant green: hay bales strewn haphazardly beneath a blazing sun. Above, the russet tussock yielded to the steeper, barer slopes— already shadowing to lavender in the slant of afternoon light. High, high above, the rocky, sunlit summits dreamed in another realm.

I gazed into a large paddock next to the cattle yards while I waited for Jim to turn up. A group of fat Hereford cows reclined at the far end, a picture of peace. Their rich red coats contrasted with the brilliant green of fresh grass resurgent above remnant wisps of hay. I love these scenes, but this was no time for reverie. Jim soon arrived in his Landrover, with a tangle of dogs on the back.

"Gidday, John."

"Where are these cows, Jim?" I asked.

"Right in front of you!" I looked more closely at the group and realised things were not as restful as they seemed. We drove up to them. Two or three of the cows were in deep respiratory stress and heaving as they fought for each breath. One cow was dead. If it was what I thought it was, I had never seen it before; indeed, it had never previously been recorded in New Zealand. The paddock had, as I had observed, been cut quite recently for hay. The old fashioned English term for the delicate tips of new grass springing up after the hay has been harvested is "foggage". Fog fever was, from my memories of fifth year veterinary medicine, typically seen in Hereford cattle released onto foggage. It is, in essence, a severe anaphylactic reaction to a chemical component (L-tryptophan) found in such pastures.

"When did you put these cows in this paddock, Jim?"

"I just let them in this morning. I lost six in here last week, but I never phoned you because I just thought it was bloat. A good thing I looked in on them just before I rang you. What do you think it is?"

I told him about fog fever. "…but to confirm it I ought to post mortem this old girl and see what her lungs look like."

We drove all the cows that we could move out of the hay paddock and onto some rough grazing. For the most severely affected of the remaining cows, struggling for breath and wheezing, I tried what I could

181

find in my car—antihistamines and even some vials of expired adrenalin. It wasn't as though you geared up in case you might run into a massive outbreak of a disease previously unrecorded in New Zealand. I was three quarters of an hour from base so, if what I had didn't work, it would take too long to obtain more.

Jim watched as I opened up the dead cow's chest with my post-mortem knife and snapped back a few ribs to expose the lungs. It's rewarding to be able to demonstrate these things to farmers. They have usually butchered meat for the house and have a fair idea of what normal organs should look like. The lungs I showed Jim were not the normal light, pink and fluffy—but heavy, waterlogged, and darkened with congested blood. Some parts had overcompensated and were stretched with emphysema. There was extensive bleeding throughout. It was easy to see that no drugs could have reversed this severe damage nor, by way of confirmation, did they seem to be making much difference to the cows I had treated earlier. However, in the end Jim was lucky and my records reveal that he only lost a couple more cows from this episode.

Hugh Montgomery, one of the veterinary pathologists at Invermay Animal Health laboratory, confirmed my suspicions from the lung sample I sent to the laboratory: Histological examination of the lungs of the dead cow showed *severe intra-alveolar oedema with a highly eosinophilic fluid in which were formed hyaline membranes and fibrin balls… Clinically and pathologically this is typical of 'fog fever'…* Hugh later submitted an article about this case concluding: *The name 'fog fever' is not related to atmospheric conditions, but derives from the British rural term 'foggage' for the regrowth occurring on paddocks cut for hay or silage. It is an unfortunate name as there is*

no fever either, but the alternative is the cumbersome
American name of 'acute bovine pulmonary oedema
and emphysema'...

~

It was the very quirkiness of the name "fog fever" that
led me to its diagnosis. Acute bovine pulmonary
oedema and emphysema (aka ABPE or bovine atypical
interstitial pneumonia) is described in modern
textbooks—but the academics still haven't managed to
dislodge that inaccurate, but memorable term "fog
fever", and I hope they never will. When diseases of
livestock have all been reduced to acronyms: SMEDI,
BVD, BHM, BSE and any other combination of capital
letters you could possibly think of, is ABPE any help?
The surfeit of acronyms favoured by modern
pathologists and clinicians merely serves to fog our
cluttered minds and pucker our fevered brows. Indeed, I
suspect that acronyms are a leading cause of human fog
fever syndrome (HUFFS).

Should this powerful plea for retaining the poetry
of our language, even into scientific matters, not have
convinced you otherwise, I would like to present
another moving story of death and dying—not of an
animal, but of a word:

A requiem for swingletrees

On one of the first farms I visited in my new career as a
vet, an old Taranaki farmer proudly demonstrated to me
his contraption for lifting a cast cow. He had linked his
Bagshaw hoist—comprising pipe-metal loops that are
tightened across the pelvis (now usually called hip
clamps) and provide the means to lift the back end of a

cow—to a stout wooden spar with a metal pivot in the centre. To the other end of the spar he had tied a thick rope in a double bowline round the cow's chest and front legs. When he raised the spar by the pivot with the front-end-loader of his tractor the cow was raised front and back. That was the theory; but in practice his contraption wasn't very efficient. If a cow isn't ready to stand she will slump, whatever high tech device is used.

My farmer's creation was a triumph of nostalgia over practicality. How disappointed he was that even I, a recent immigrant from the "old country", didn't know what that wooden spar was called. It was, in fact, a sturdy relic from the days of horse power: a *swingletree* (also, delightfully, a whippletree).

As a lad he had harnessed up the family Clydesdale to a cart or plough using that swingletree, securing the traces at each end to the collar of his massive companion, and bolting the plough through the pivot. This arrangement permitted a straight pull and eliminated the tendency for the plough to see-saw at each stride. Alas, in me, my farmer was dealing with a generation profoundly ignorant of what had once been a major part of his life. The horse, in agriculture, has all but gone. But, more insidiously, an ancient vocabulary is vanishing with it.

And now it is my turn to mourn. For in the very word swingletree I sense a route to Old English that will soon fade into oblivion. William Langland's pious character, Piers Plowman, one of the first men to walk the pages of mediaeval English literature, would have been able to share my old farmer's dreams, as would all the generations over more than seven hundred years since; yet I could not. New words may come thick and fast, replacing those we lose—modem, router, i-pod, javascript—but without the historical links they seem disconnected and ephemeral. They weren't here yesterday and they won't be here tomorrow. They lack the life force of swingletrees, hames and crupper straps—although I did feel something very powerful was going on when the "motherboard" recently crashed my computer!

Chapter Twenty-one

Music for Cows: Radios for Racing

Music is said to be the speech of angels: in fact, nothing among the utterances allowed to man is felt to be so divine. It brings us near to the infinite. – Thomas Carlyle (1795-1881)

It is not a good idea to rely on the newspapers for unbiased and useful scientific information. Sometimes, however, it would be nice if it were. I would love to believe the reports I read about music played to animals as a form of relaxation—something that makes cows more settled in the shed, pigs more porky and hens more clucky. It is a touchy-feely subject and I know of no scientific proof that it works. Conclusive proof of well-being for animal scientists tends to be linked to increased productivity, which is a measurable effect: higher milk yields, faster weight gains, more eggs. Happiness per se, is not measurable. But a happy cow, the theory goes, will produce more milk than a sad cow. Currently, cows are not amenable to brain scans; however, someday in the future the technology will be found and we will then be able to monitor their happiness directly.

   Usually the type of music recommended to increase milk production is classical in style. To me this is rational. Cows are, in the main, serene animals. They respond to serene owners. The cows in a shed which is soothed by the cheerful elegance of baroque music are likely to release more milk than one blaring with angry rap. But this could be an indirect effect. The chances are that the staff who listen to classical music are more likely to be at peace with themselves than those revved up by a barrage of violence or hatred.

In fact linkages between the temperament of the staff who handle cows and cow health have been irrefutably proven in studies of lameness. The milker who habitually rushes cows to the shed, anxious that they don't intrude on his night in the pub, will have more lame cows than the placid farmer who patiently drifts his herd to milking while ignoring the fuming motorist stuck behind him.

An experienced and observant vet will pick up on such subtleties. The farmer whose dogs are open and friendly is generally better to deal with than he who owns the timid, retiring kind—often a sign of abuse. Likewise, if I was to turn up at a previously unknown cow shed and had the choice of dealing with a shed hand emerging from a background of orchestral music or one who stepped from a pit of snarling guitars and adenoidal vowels, I am sure that my prejudices, as you now see them emerging, would be validated.

The post war generation, to which I belong, has seen many innovations and technological advances which have immeasurably improved our lives. However, music seems to be the one area where we have lost ground. My upbringing was largely in the pre-television era. Some of my earliest memories are invoked by the music on the radio to which I was exposed in early childhood. "Listen with Mother" was an institution in the 1950s. The beautifully enunciated: "Are you sitting comfortably? Then I'll begin" was heralded by the delightfully wistful Berceuse from Fauré's Dolly Suite though, of course, I didn't know this at the time. By contrast, our present failure to enhance children's emotional development through exposure to music of eloquence and beauty passes unremarked. Indeed, the absence of anything approaching the sublime in their lives may be one factor fuelling an inappropriate search for it later in life via alcoholism and drug abuse.

Light orchestral music was frequently played on the radio throughout my childhood and my ear gained an appreciation, which in my case later evolved into a passion for serious classical music. If music is the food of love, it was certainly a catalyst in my developing relationship with the lovely young lady I was courting, who would later become my wife. Viv and I both share the same tastes in music. While the psychologists claim that the initial period when a couple are actually "in love" lasts only one year, they neglect the power of great music. Truly great music has the ability to move and inspire the soul, and summon feelings akin to those we feel when we are in love. We are reborn and refreshed. Under the influence of sublime music the sublime is possible.

For anyone raised in Liverpool during the 1960s, my musical proclivities may seem strange. The "Beatles" must surely feature somewhere? Well yes, they do. I used to cycle every day to school around the side of a large open park named "The Mystery", cross busy Smithfield Road and then on, down a narrower street which passed a fire station and then humped over a railway line—steep for a bicycle—and eventually came out alongside our school playing fields.

As I grew older, I noted that the solid British-Empire-quality, cast-iron signage for this narrow street regularly disappeared. It was in an accessible position bolted into wooden pegs in a low sandstone wall. The "Penny Lane" sign was obviously a desirable acquisition and soon the city council gave up replacing it. Rathbone Hall, a university hall of residence, was opposite. I suspect that Penny Lane signs now grace the walls of respectable middle-class abodes belonging to some former Rathbone Hall residents. They will endure long after the tatty Che Guevera posters of their youth have peeled away. Penny Lane was my closest link with the Beatles—but their tuneful music was everywhere during my later school years and we all waited for their next hit.

The Beatles were not universally approved. An older generation condemned them as "long-haired layabouts". The peacefully stable society for which they had fought during two world wars was under threat. At school, rigorous attention was paid to the cardinal sins: wearing trousers without turn-ups, or having hair less than an inch above the collar. Few got away with flouting the "short back and sides" rule.

Peter Callaghan got away with it for a while by using wallpaper paste, but his scheme fell badly awry one wet and windy day. He was doing his duty as a compulsory supporter on the sidelines for a school first XV rugby match when a patrolling master spotted him:

"Callaghan, what have you done with your hair?"

"Nothing sir."

"Then why is it snaking down over your collar?"

"I don't know, sir."

"Don't be ridiculous, boy. And what is that revolting muck you've put in it? Report for detention tomorrow evening with your hair cut and properly washed!"

"Yes, sir." With which Callaghan was brought down to size (not of the wallpaper variety) and consigned to an hour of vigorous physical exercise after school under the supervision of some vindictive prefect.

But Beetlemania was merely the unimportant outward sign of what some would see as a deeper moral disintegration of society. The birth control pill was transforming sexual mores and the increasing abuses of recreational drugs were more major concerns. Many of the older generation shut their ears to the music of the Beatles because they saw them and their ilk as champions of the new decadence. In vain I importuned my parents to open their hearts: the Beatles were tuneful and inventive. But my pleas were cast on flinty ground. Why? I argued; their private lives were no worse than those of the great composers. Tchaikovsky was a homosexual, Beethoven an alcoholic who died of liver disease, Wagner an adulterer, Erik Satie an alcoholic who dabbled in the occult, Percy Grainger enjoyed a good spanking, Schubert was a hedonistic syphilitic, Smetana a deaf syphilitic, Delius a syphilitic who went blind and, worst of all, Sir Edward Elgar was a Roman Catholic! To this day they remain obdurate: the Beatles pioneered the downfall of decent society. The way things have turned out, perhaps they had a point. But, if we look behind the smokescreens, when was there ever a truly decent society? My parents' generation's supposedly decent, post-war society accepted the suppression of women, and was indulging in an orgy of institutionalised child abuse that wouldn't be uncovered for decades. There is always a dark side to human nature whether we choose to acknowledge it or sweep it under the mat.

The Beatles remain a mere footnote in my story of musical appreciation. I was always impelled to follow music that fed my soul and which has led me on a life-long journey of exploration. "Mull of Kintyre" didn't quite do that for me, but my early encounter with Fauré triggered something that I fear has been denied to today's children raised on a diet of commercial radio. Music which so beautifully expresses feelings of poignancy, joy, excitement, sorrow, and yearning has been denied them as the English speaking world largely seems to have turned its back on classical music and prefers to embrace each new day with the yap of commercial radio. It's one thing to choose to atrophy your temporal lobes in the privacy of your own home, but quite another to afflict your tastes on all and sundry. I certainly was not prepared to tolerate it in my own work place.

For several days after my appointment as senior vet at Otautau I put up with the radio that our receptionist played in the clinic. I frequently returned from my rounds as "Humpy" or "Woody" or "Boggy" or some other "----y" announced the winners of the "----quizznite", or a crass trumpet fanfare heralded a commercial for farmers (deep gravely voice) or twittered on about the new washing powder available at "xzy, jingle, jingle"—repeated three times.

In my opinion the playing of commercial radio in shops and waiting rooms is deplorable and so, politely, I asked our receptionist to desist. She had the grace to do so most of the time, but occasionally I would arrive back from my rounds and there was an important horse race running and the two to one favourite was backing a trifecta [or whatever] at the Trentham derby and they're off in that staccato manner that anyone not interested in racing can't understand but finds intensely irritating because it keeps on rasping away without a pause so that you cannot ignore it... last furlong to go and it's Smegma from Borborygmi... Smegma from Borborygmi... Smegma from Borborygmi and Smegma takes it by a length from Borborygmi then followed two lengths back by Butcher's Fart with Mindless Spree the favourite finishing last... But at last it winds down and you are ready to collect your winnings on Smegma or

191

some other silly effing name before race two and the cycle is going to begin again. Racing! And we're off ...

"For goodness sake turn that thing off, S~, how many times do I have to tell you? How can you serve customers while you're listening to that crap?"

"Orrrh John! Just because you aren't interested in racing. My uncle's got a starter in race five."

S~'s love affair with the radio at the clinic suddenly ended when it mysteriously died and no-one was able to revive it. After that the reception area remained unpolluted by radio. Of course, we could have purchased a hi-fi system and filled our rooms with music, but whenever the topic was resurrected there was considerable debate as to exactly what music should be played. We never reached a consensus. Silence reigned! It seems the pleasure to be derived from listening to music you enjoy is likely to be outweighed by the displeasure incurred from being compelled to listen to something you hate.

~

Over the years I have seen many young vets start on their daily rounds entombed in cars reverberating to thumping, jarring rhythms. That is their look-out, but I'm sure that we're not that different from dairy cows and that everyone would be happier and more productive if they were exposed to classical music. Unfortunately, compulsory exposure to music, even of the highest quality, defeats the object. Perhaps we should reverse our thinking and adopt recent anti-smoking tactics and condemn undesirable listening habits. If the link with poor mental health could be established we could then legislate for warning signs to be placed on CDs of degenerate music: "C & W music may be intellectually debilitating", or "Rap kills".

At the same time the use of earphones would be made mandatory to protect the rest of us from the dangers of passive listening. It is socially unacceptable.

Before my pen gets too carried away on this wave of hyperbole, I have to remind myself that some of my best friends enjoy heavy metal (despite me imploring them that lead and mercury are toxic) and one, even, speaks favourably of Johnny Cash. To misquote Mrs Campbell: what care I so long as they don't play it in the milking parlour and frighten the cows.

Chapter Twenty-two

The Holistic Approach

Prevention is so much better than healing, because it saves the labour of being sicke. – T Adams (1618)

By the early 1990s many North Island dairy farmers were attracted to Southland by cheaper land. The first wave established Southland's potential as a Mecca for dairying and the trickle of farms converting from sheep into dairying became close to a flood. It wasn't all plain sailing for these pioneers as they adjusted to a new life. Moving farm is not as straightforward as moving house.

Thousands of cows were trucked down from the Waikato and Taranaki onto Southland's green pastures. Many arrived lame and injured from their long journeys until the trucking firms realised that a careful driver generated fewer insurance claims than a careless one. A fast driver with a good record for turn around times was, in the long run, an expensive liability. A slow, smooth driver delivered his charges relatively uninjured. These dairying families were coming to newly built milking sheds, newly fenced paddocks and newly established lanes for movement of stock around the farm. Some arrived to find the milking shed wasn't finished, the fencing was only half done and the river gravel used to metal the lanes was totally unsuitable and injuring their cows' feet.

It was not unusual for vets to be called to attend a dozen or more lame and injured cows that had just come off a truck. You might arrive to find them in a paddock with no yards and therefore no means of restraining them for treatment. What are you going to

194

do? You're the vet, I've called you out to do the job, so get to it. Usually some unsatisfactory compromise could be sorted out which would reinforce the fact that you were not half as good as their old vets back home.

I was greeted on one of these new farms by this familiar refrain: "We used to use old Whatnot. Have you heard of him? Best dairy vet in the Waikato. Of course, you're not used to dealing with dairy cows down here are you?" … etcetera.

Perhaps we were unduly sensitive, but being told you're second best before you've even begun is either irritating or depressing—depending on how your day has been. I got out my deer pole—that surprised him, he'd never seen one of those before—and I was able to inject the injured cows in the paddock. Cows are not stupid. They are well aware of man's never-ending quest to stick needles in them; so I had to run after one or two to get within range, but my pole gave me a longer reach than they were accustomed to—possibly further than old Whatnot's prodigious span. A few minutes later and six cows were sleeping in various parts of the paddock. Of course it was far more time-consuming to do it this way than if the farmer had the proper facilities and so his fee for my services was inevitably more than old Whatnot would have charged. We heard all about that too.

Our work was changing. We spent more and more time with stressed dairy farmers adjusting to new farms, new neighbours, new financial pressures, new schools for their children—and us, their new vets. It was good for veterinary business, but something of the old harmony was gone. The whole rural community, once reassuringly immutable, had been destabilised.

In early June each year there is now a "gipsy day". On this one day of the year a large number of dairy farmers play "musical farms" and move to occupy another property. For twenty-four hours the roads are a madness of plodding cows and desperate stockmen. School rolls change overnight and vets re-align their lists of clients and wait to see which of the new mix of gentlefolk and psychopaths will emerge to seek their help.

All this time, as Sid drove on his rounds, his mind was awhirl with the calculations so necessary to his advisory work. He would arrive back to inform us that we could expect trouble on X's new conversion.

"There's 1200 kgs of dry matter over the farm and he's got 425 cows going onto 200 hectares and they're only about condition score 4. I think he's asking for trouble at this time of year. He's going to have to buy in supplements. What do you reckon, John?"

The trouble with geniuses like Sid is that they fail to recognise mathematical dyslexia in people like me. I could never have asked the question, still less given an answer. I may well have observed that the cows were thin, that the stockman wore a lean and hungry look, that his dog cowered when his master looked his way and that there was quite a lot of ragwort in some of the paddocks—I would even write a newspaper article about that. But putting it in numbers? Given the same situation Giles would have noticed the new raceways were poorly engineered with insufficient drainage fall which could cause lameness, that there was insufficient vacuum reserve in the milking plant X had installed and that with his hi-line system he was asking for mastitis. Daryl would have found out that X was a bit of bastard really, but he was a keen hunter and he (Daryl) had already arranged to go out and give the whole herd copper bullets the next day.

Working as a team the four of us, with our disparate skills, were able to offer a comprehensive service to these assertive new dairy farmers. For the first milking season after their move there were often meaty animal health issues for us to get our teeth into as they and their cows adjusted to their new farm.

DD was one of these new dairy farmers and some, like him, seemed to have continuing problems, even though we had corrected some basic trace-element deficiencies. It took a couple of years of detective work to get to the bottom of it.

Firstly, he seemed to have more than his fair share of calves born dead, or dying soon after birth. Later in spring some of his cows became sick and some of these died, too. All our post-mortems and tests failed to reveal a common cause. There is little to observe in the carcases of cows dying from metabolic diseases, especially if they die in the night unseen, with no telltale symptoms. No doubt some of these deaths were metabolic. We found nothing remarkable on autopsy, save the odd liver abscess. Since these are quite a common finding, we did not attach much significance to them.

As summer hardens into autumn, the dairy farmer takes note of his least productive cows. He cannot afford to carry passengers, and he requires that every mouth eating his grass turns it into milk as efficiently as possible. He draws up a list of cows he needs to cull. They include those which have chronic untreatable diseases such as mastitis or arthritis, cows which have failed to get in calf and cows which, for some reason, are thin and fail to milk as well as they should. DD had a lot of these. They went for slaughter, their trimmed remains lingering in manufacturing grade meats exported to far away places. But many of DD's culls

197

did not even make it to the world's pizza parlours and hamburger bars: many were failing to pass meat inspection. The killing-sheet reports revealed another piece of the puzzle. These cows were rejected because they had liver abscesses. More to the point, DD was not alone. It was quite a common problem for the whole dairy industry in the south of New Zealand. What was going on?

Sid was concerned about DD's heavy reliance on brassica crops to feed his cows through winter. Those of you who abhor cabbages, broccoli, kale, or swedes will perhaps understand why they can, sometimes, be regarded as noxious. It has long been recognised that brassicas contain chemicals poisonous to livestock and must be fed with care. As cattle food they are low in fibre, low in trace elements such as selenium and copper, and they are full of polyunsaturated fatty acids that reduce the availability of fat soluble vitamins such as vitamin E. None of these things excuse children turning up their noses at a helping of these useful vegetables; but if they were the sole component of their diets, well that would be a different matter. DD's cows, like many others in Southland, were fed nothing but kale for several weeks before they calved.

Sid tested some of them for vitamin E: a very expensive test and seldom used for this very reason. DD's cows registered the lowest detectable levels. Calves born to such cows were bound to be deficient in this vital nutrient. We had a possible explanation for the unexplained calf deaths.

Sid's next stroke of intuition came from his interest in the workings of the rumen, the vast vat that is the first of the four stomachs of a cow. Here a seething multitude of micro-organisms break down the ingested vegetation in a process akin to garden composting. And, just as for the garden compost heap, the mix of fibre to greens is important. If fibre is lacking in the diet, the process veers out of balance. If the rumen contents become too acidic, they set off a chain of undesirable consequences. The acids eat at the lining of the rumen and the vague and fluctuating symptoms of this digestive upset manifest as a general malaise, lack of appetite and diarrhoea: a vague syndrome known as "acidosis". The acid damage to the rumen wall renders it permeable. Bacteria-laden fluid can now leak into the circulation and colonise other organs of the body.

The liver is the first major organ to receive the inflow of blood from a cow's stomachs. Normally, this blood is enriched by molecules of broken-down nutrients, ready for the Krebs' cycle biochemical processes in which the liver specialises. Unfortunately, in these acidotic cows, the blood also bears a cargo of pathogenic bacteria. The immune system struggles to eliminate these bugs, and the white cells in the blood, losing their fight, die in millions—forming the pus we had seen as liver abscesses. The body tries to wall this battlefield of dead cells and bacteria behind layers of fibrous tissue: abscesses. Internal abscesses like these cannot be drained like a skin boil, neither can antibiotics reach the bacteria within their enclosing walls. Occasionally the walling-in is effective; the bacteria are contained, and the cow recovers—her blemished, battle scarred liver revealed only at slaughter. More usually, the bacteria periodically burst through the abscess walls and invade more liver tissue, causing further debilitation. They may even spread into the abdominal cavity causing a localised, or even a generalised, peritonitis. Such cows suffer constant cycles of ill health, yet they occur at intervals so far removed from the initial faulty diet that its role in their illness or death is not obvious. Liver abscesses have causes other than acidosis, obscuring the link with the faulty diet even further. These days every cattle farmer realises the importance of feeding extra fibre, in the form of hay or straw, to balance out the diet when they are feeding brassicas.

We knew it would take time for DD's herd health to recover. Some of his cows would be sequentially debilitated by their liver episodes for years before they finally succumbed. But DD was still not entirely happy. Even the young cows, which should have benefited from his improved winter feeding regimen, were not milking as well as they should. Further blood sampling suggested that his cows always tended to be slightly dehydrated. By this stage we had been working with John Scandrett, a farm consultant who was an expert in soils and was looking at DD's effluent disposal system. He obtained a flow meter and monitored how much the cows were drinking. The answer, in short, was not enough.

The reason, as we found out, was that the water was iron rich. This encouraged the growth of unpalatable bacteria. The cows did not like its taste. When DD installed a UV purifying system and clean water was filling his water troughs, his cows increased their milk output almost overnight.

In the veterinary world, many of the simple, one-fix problems have been solved. The dramatic improvement in herd health throughout much of New Zealand following the widespread use of trace element supplements had created an unrealistic faith that other tonics could solve complex problems at a stroke. In comparable situations to DD's, other farmers have wasted years tipping expensive and ineffective supplements down the throats of their stock.

Unravelling the reasons for his poorly producing herd was a fascinating journey involving teamwork with other experts from whom we all learned a great deal. Along the way there were many frustrations, usually associated with the costs of the investigations, particularly when they seemed to be going nowhere. In the end the findings were of benefit to many other farmers and farm consultants.

In agriculture, as in many other fields of human endeavour, the giant strides are few and far between. Progress is often by the small, unheralded steps of competent people working cooperatively.

~

Larry, the manager of a sheep farm, had taken delivery of several hundred lambs from a high country station. He planned to fatten them on his rich low-lying pastures. It had been a wet spring and, although it was muddy, he had plenty of grass to feed their hungry mouths. The lambs disembarked from the stock trucks and into his muddy yards where they were weighed and drenched for worms. They were a bit thin, but he fully expected them to pile on weight before too long. He flung open his gates and loosed them in large mobs and watched with satisfaction as they tucked into the best feed they had ever seen.

The wet weather continued. The lambs, which had at first picked up, were now less perky. They started to lose condition. Some started scouring and some died. Larry brought in a few of the dead lambs and from some of them the laboratory grew a nasty bacterium, *Listeria ivanovii*. Bacteria of the genus *Listeria* can cause severe gut infections (and are frequently associated with food poisoning in humans). They are also responsible for abortions in animals and women. But, of the species *ivanovii*, not a lot was known— except it was suspected to be a problem in wet conditions.

Modern society has, until very recently, placed great faith in the power of antibiotics to fight disease and, faced with outbreaks of infection, there still is the temptation to mass medicate and treat the whole flock. We considered it, but these days there is greater awareness of the risks of such blunderbuss approaches, especially regarding the development of antibiotic resistance. Pastoral farming systems have not, for the most part, been tainted by this sort of misuse of drugs, although it has been common in housed animal, factory farming systems—especially with pigs and poultry. Besides, since *Listeria* can hang around in the environment, any benefit from mass medication on Larry's farm would probably be temporary and the cost high.

Sid and I visited the farm to see what was going on. Many of the paddocks were muddy. Larry had noticed that the lamb mobs were walking in circles and making matters worse by trampling the grass into the mud. It was this observation, plus the results of an analysis of puddle water—the only water available to these lambs—which led us to an explanation for their poor performance. Lambs need clean food and water. Because the paddocks were large, the lambs were being left in them for several days rather than being moved onto fresh, clean grass each day. This would have been fine in dry conditions, but in the wet they were tramping their food into the mud. They were circling restlessly because they were in search of clean food. The term faecal-oral transmission probably requires no explanation. Mud wasn't the only foreign matter garnishing their diet.

Normally, in wet conditions, lambs don't drink much, there being sufficient water in their grass diet. However many of these lambs had enteritis, lambs with diarrhoea drink more, and the only source of water was from the puddles. Our tests revealed that these puddles contained coliform counts of over four thousand per ml, far above the acceptable limit of less than 100. The bore water on the same farm had a count of 12, so plenty of clean water was available, albeit at a price.

The long-term solution for this farm lay not in drugs. Larry needed to subdivide the paddocks, so that the lambs could be moved more frequently onto fresh, clean grass. He needed to set up a system of water troughs so that they had access to clean water. Money also needed to be spent improving the drainage system across the farm. Good management is a far better way of preventing disease than masking poor management by misusing drugs. Unfortunately, the overheads involved in farming are little appreciated by the general public.

~

Why would I choose to exemplify these two cases? Perhaps it is to show how the involvement of the veterinary profession in farming has changed over the years: years when the public's perception of what it does has lagged several decades behind the reality. The emphasis has moved away from treatment of individual animals, to a more holistic consideration of the farm itself; from the losses due to clinical disease, to the hidden effects of sub-clinical diseases (diseases which produce no overt signs of their presence) on the productivity of the herd or flock; from intervention to prevention. We now have a much better idea of how healthy, well-fed farm animals should perform and what "best practice" procedures to put in place to attain optimum productivity.

It's a far cry from the early years of the profession, 250 years ago.

Chapter Twenty-three

Foot and Mouth, and the Detritus Gene

Mr Sutton said the Reserve Bank had estimated the impact of a foot and mouth disease outbreak here as costing about $6 billion in GDP in the first year and about $10 billion in GDP in the second year. "So, it's a hugely important area, and it's crucial that everyone – individuals and groups – work together to ensure the response is as integrated and comprehensive as possible." – Government release from the Minister of Biosecurity, Jim Sutton, April 2005.

Veterinarians, in the 1790s were scarcely better than the quacks they were trying to displace. In 1897, in *The Veterinary Record*, William Hunting writing about the advances of the previous sixty years, still felt that the high position that the veterinary profession had attained during Victoria's reign only marked "its arrival at adolescence". He noted: *In 1837 every wretched animal that was submitted to veterinary treatment underwent a course of bleeding, physicing and blistering ... Professor Sewell asserted that bad feeling and ill usage might cause rabies in dogs ... everyone believed that a healthy sign was... when a wound 'mattered freely' ... men with the mere ability to read and write with difficulty could enter the ranks... twelve months study was all that was demanded.*

The Professor Sewell to whom William Hunting referred was obviously a controversial figure. It was Sewell who had, notoriously, prescribed ridiculous treatments for the new vesicular disease of cattle which made its appearance near London in 1839. This disease was, in fact, foot and mouth (FMD). Professor Sewell's recommended treatment regimen (for a disease as untreatable now as it was then) included the usual catalogue of harmful intrusions: copper sulphate for the sore mouths and feet, blisters and bleeding, soda and ginger, calomel, and setons in the throat or dewlap. (Setons were loops of twine or tape sewn through the skin to encourage suppuration).

A survey by the secretary of the Royal College of Veterinary Surgeons in 1848 which sought to categorise all the various people treating animals revealed that *...under the various denominations of horse-doctors, horse-surgeons, farriers, cowleeches, cattle-doctors, castrators, spayers and gelders, charmers, spell-workers, butty-colliers, water-doctors, and various other local appellations, those who gain a livelihood by the practice of the art... far exceeded those who had been to veterinary school.* But perhaps, had Professor Sewell taught them, their veterinary training would have conferred little benefit to their patients in these early years.

Showmanship came first. There must have been a marvellous sense of theatre about these bold treatments. After all, those Victorian vets had to impress if they were to elicit payment from stingy farmers and hard-bitten horsemen. It was not what you did, but how you did it—a lesson that is as relevant to new veterinary graduates today as it was then. No wonder if some of the public turned to far less injurious alternatives such as homeopathy, even if they, too, were ineffective. However, by the middle of the century, men of scientific integrity were starting to appear.

The year 1865 (the very year Carl Volkner was murdered at Opotiki) finally showed the worth of a profession starting to embrace Pasteur's research and understand the role of animalcules (micro-organisms) in the spread of disease. That is the year Cattle Plague (Rinderpest), thought to have been imported from Russia, killed an estimated half million cattle in Britain. It was only halted when veterinary measures—advocated but not adopted at the beginning—were finally put in place. Those who promoted the older theory of "spontaneous generation" which maintained that diseases appeared out of thin air—such as Viscount Cranbourne—were finally over-ruled. In Victorian Britain, things were always trickier if the aristocracy were not on your side. In the end, science prevailed and the Animal Health Division of the Ministry of Agriculture was established.

Cattle Plague/ Rinderpest, the most severe infectious disease of cattle the world has ever known, was finally eradicated in 2011. This, by amazing coincidence, was the sestercentennial year since the founding of the veterinary profession by Louis XV in 1761, specifically to eliminate Cattle Plague.

Unfortunately, there are many other threats: like FMD. Control of such highly infectious diseases remains the chief responsibility of the veterinary profession and it is the reason behind the continued government funding of veterinary education. The worst mistake a veterinary practitioner could ever make would be to miss a diagnosis of an "exotic disease" and place the whole agricultural economy of his country at risk. For New Zealand, where the largest portion of the country's gross domestic product is generated by pastoral industries, the consequences of such a miss would be catastrophic. Vets in New Zealand have long proven their worth. As long ago as 1880 Messrs Richie and Naden eradicated a deadly outbreak of bovine pleuropneumonia in the Waikato. What would it be like to carry the blame for an error of judgement in Southland in 1981 that had the potential to break the entire economy of New Zealand?

Thoughts like these accompanied me as I drove out to Jack's pig farm. Jack only had a couple of breeding sows and one of them had sores on its teats. Such a call-out would not, in the normal course of events, have raised my blood pressure. But this particular morning it did. The reason was that another pig farm near Temuka, a couple of hundred kilometres to the north of us, was currently at the centre of an FMD emergency. The whole of New Zealand was on a full scale alert because the pigs at Temuka had blisters on their feet and snouts and were under investigation by MAF. Movement controls were in force and samples had been sent to Pirbright, a laboratory in England specialising in FMD, for testing. The daily TV news was milking it for all it was worth. The economic future of New Zealand hung in the balance. Well done the vet who had raised the alarm! He had not failed in his line of duty.

I knew that teat blisters could occur in pigs with FMD, although there would also be lesions on the snout and, possibly, the feet as well. Jack hadn't mentioned these, but then he didn't have a lot of experience of pig farming, having come to it as a self-sufficiency project late in life.

Jack led "The Good Life" on the couple of muddy acres surrounding his dilapidated weatherboard house. There never seems to be a shortage of used wire mattress frames, broken prams or discarded refrigerators to patch up the fence holes on small-scale pig operations such as his; for Jack belonged to that sub-tribe of mankind who possess the "detritus" gene and are thereby rendered oblivious to their surroundings. They spend all their weekends and holidays at the local rubbish dump—battered flat-deck ute and recycled trailer at the ready—fossicking for free in their second-hand tea-cosy hats, soiled dungarees and holey gumboots. And a lifestyle which for me, and many others, would have presaged a bleak and sordid descent into old age, for Jack offered a treasure trove of beady-eyed opportunity: to save, scrimp and scrounge.

Pigs are not easy to examine, even in the best of facilities. In my mind's eye I pictured crawling through a filthy, bodged-up pen of rotting, tip-salvaged doors to examine my new patient—just as I had on previous visits.

FMD outbreaks often start in pigs. They are highly susceptible to the virus and it rapidly multiplies once it infects them. Pig farms then become virus "factories" from which plumes of infection arise and are spewed downwind. The virus can jump many miles like this, in addition to being carried by people, vehicles, on contaminated stockfeed and, of course, on and within transported animals.

As I drove to Jack's, I imagined what I would do if I found the sow with sore teats also had tell-tale vesicles (blisters) on her snout and round her feet, a raised temperature, and was starting to smack her lips and salivate as the sores made their presence felt. The correct procedures to follow in the event of a suspected diagnosis of FMD had been thoroughly inculcated in me on the "exotic disease" training courses I had attended a few years earlier. I checked my glove compartment to find the little card with the number of the MAF vet I would have to ring the moment I suspected the worst. I planned where I would park my car at the entrance to Jack's drive to stop all movement on or off the premises. There were sure to be a couple of rusting fridges and a twisted trampoline or two to reinforce the barricade. And should my investigations reveal any hint of the presence of FMD on the farm there was the delightful prospect of being confined there for several days of squalor with the genial but disorganised Jack. It didn't hold much appeal.

My reveries were broken by a voice on the RT. "Vet base to vet 11".

"Go ahead Audrey."

"Jack has just rung to say he doesn't need a vet any more. His neighbour reckons it's just due to the sharp teeth of the piglets she's suckling."

I did not feel any immediate sense of relief. What if the neighbour was wrong? Was it still Jack's decision? I chewed it over.

"OK Audrey, but I'll have to discuss it with the RVO [Regional Veterinary Officer] to decide what to do next."

In the event, and much to my relief, the RVO assumed responsibility. So Jack was untroubled by my presence, but perhaps a little surprised when the RVO turned up just to confirm how much damage a suckling piglet can do to mum with those sharp little nippers.

Better to be safe than sorry—about the pigs and the national economy, that is. As to the RVO, soon after this incident he left his job in Invercargill for a more exotic location in the Pacific Islands. It would be idle to speculate, but perhaps the move was expedited by his encounter with Jack and the detritus gene.

The Temuka outbreak was interesting. No FMD virus was isolated from the affected pigs. Despite the blisters, they remained healthy and never ran fevers. The conclusion was that this was a case of parsnip poisoning. A similar condition had been reported among horticulture workers handling celery or parsnips, which, like some other umbelliferous plants, contain chemicals called *furocoumarins* in their leaves. These are absorbed into the skin and react with sunlight, releasing energy that damages the skin cells—hence the blistering. All that is required is the combination of pigs, parsnips and sunlight of a particular wavelength. The pathology of the disease was not clarified until the early 1980s—which only goes to show that there is always something new under the sun.

FMD is an excellent illustration of why the New Zealand government should do all it can to preserve a vigilant veterinary presence throughout its rural hinterland.

I remain eternally grateful that during my career as a farm vet I have never been involved with a genuine outbreak of FMD in New Zealand. If one should ever occur, the stresses for all concerned will be truly enormous.

Chapter Twenty-four

Science and Drama

*... slight disturbances precipitate attacks of
continuous bellowing and frenzied galloping. The gait
becomes staggering and the animal falls with obvious
tetany of the limbs which is rapidly followed by clonic
convulsions lasting for about a minute. During these
convulsive episodes there is opisthotonus, nystagmus,
champing of the jaws, frothing at the mouth, pricking of
the ears, and retraction of the eyelids. Between
episodes the animal lies quietly, but a sudden noise or
touch may precipitate another attack. The temperature
rises after severe muscle exertion... the absolute
intensity of the heart sounds is increased so that they
can be heard some distance away from the cow. Death
usually occurs within half to one hour and the mortality
rate is high because many die before treatment can be
provided...* from *Veterinary Medicine*. Third Edition,
1968: Blood and Henderson

With this classic description of grass staggers in cattle,
I salute a moment of high drama from the pages of
Blood and Henderson, a textbook venerated by
generations of vets and veterinary undergraduates, and
more remembered for the apt name of one of its authors
than its rather forgettable title. Large tracts of
veterinary textbooks date as rapidly as scientific
knowledge expands; but vivid descriptions of the
presenting signs of most diseases remain valid for as
long as they exist.

During my life as a veterinarian, science
unravelled many of the mysteries of animal health.

Practising vets, not just those who work in research, are in a great position to contribute to this body of knowledge. It is the duty of every vet not merely to treat and cure but, where possible, to investigate the underlying causes of anything unusual that comes his, or her, way—most of us have degrees in veterinary *science*, after all. Furthermore, they should make every effort to have their findings published for the good of all. Only when a problem has been revealed, and its causes discovered, can effective steps be taken to mitigate its effects or prevent it happening again.

I was very fortunate in my first job in New Zealand to work under a principal who encouraged his vets to question and investigate. Hank de Jong had a research background at the Wallaceville Animal Research Centre but, after several years as a microbiologist, had been drawn back into veterinary practice. Aside from his work Hank could be absent-minded and, sometimes, impractical. These traits led to him inviting—without first asking Viv and me—a young veterinarian and his wife and their two pre-school children to stay *with us*. We had only been in New Zealand a few weeks.

It was a trying time because I was getting to grips with my new career in a strange country and Viv had just started a new job in Stratford, the neighbouring town. All our furniture and appliances were in transit from England. We were hardly in a position to play the part of gracious hosts. We were sleeping on the floor in our sleeping bags: no bed, no table and two borrowed kitchen chairs. On the other hand, this was kind-hearted Hank, who was so supportive of me, a new graduate, in my first encounters with the wild farmers of Taranaki. How could I refuse? I dreaded what Viv would think when I told her, but Hank had anticipated my mild objections and he offered to lend us some essentials, including a mattress from his open garage. The mattress smelled as though it had been a favourite lurk of the local cats and it was memorably flea ridden. I would have offended him had I refused it.

In the event everything worked out well. John and Maureen Pauli became friends in adversity and we all rattled along famously in our nearly empty house, although Viv and their children were badly affected by the flea bites.

John was doing research into hypomagnesaemia in cattle: low blood magnesium levels. These are found, most dramatically, in grass staggers. Hypomagnesaemia was a common problem on Taranaki farms during spring when the cows calved and came into milk. Cows are on a knife-edge when their magnesium levels are low and they needed only the slightest stress, if any at all—a spell of cold weather, a walk to the milking shed, another cow bullying them—to tip them into the convulsions which *Blood and Henderson* so vividly describes. It was something all farmers dreaded.

If there was any chance of saving them at this point, they needed urgent treatment. This involved infusing a magnesium solution *slowly* into the jugular vein: not the easiest thing to accomplish on a powerful beast thrashing about mindlessly. If the distracted vet—dodging flailing hooves and bent on self-preservation—ran the magnesium into the vein too rapidly, the patient could go into cardiac arrest and die. Death never looked good when it was on the end of your flutter valve needle. If the treatment was too late the animal, exhausted and with major muscle damage, would relapse into a semi-comatose state from which she would never fully recover.

There were various refinements we used to improve our success rates. Sometimes we injected small but concentrated doses of anaesthetic into the vein to stop the convulsions while the magnesium was run in, and often we diluted the magnesium solution with calcium borogluconate to lessen its impact on the heart. This made sense because hypomagnesaemia and hypocalcaemia often go hand in hand. Sometimes, if the beast was nervy and teetering on the borderline—still standing, but just on the point of going into convulsions—we would run the magnesium slowly under the skin, because just trying to restrain nervy cows in order to insert a needle in the vein was enough to tip them into full-scale threshing-machine mode, whereas if the solution was trickled under the skin with minimum restraint or stress, and the cow was left quietly alone, the magnesium would slowly take effect and calm her down. It was all a matter of clinical judgement based on experience. The emphasis, for the moments of your call-out, was on treatment, and that was where the drama lay; the interest, however, lay in the science.

John Pauli was interested in the magnesium concentrations in the cerebro-spinal fluid (CSF) of these cows. We knew that their blood serum levels were low, but what of the concentrations in the fluid surrounding the brain? How readily did magnesium cross the blood-brain barrier? If magnesium in the blood were slow to cross into the brain fluid perhaps it would explain why treatment responses were so variable.

Unfortunately, it is quite difficult to obtain CSF samples from a cow, even if it is compliant and restrained in a crush. It involves inserting a long, fine needle through the tough skin and ligaments at the back of the neck, advancing it through a gap between the atlas vertebra and the back of the skull, and tapping the fluid from a structure called the *cisterna magna*. John wanted to obtain samples of CSF from the cows *while they were convulsing*. He accompanied me on my rounds day and night hoping to see a convulsing cow and get the farmer's permission to obtain a CSF sample from it. On a few occasions we were there at the right time and, I'll never know how, he did manage to hit the cisterna magnae of several thrashing cows. As I recollect, for all his efforts, he never obtained sufficient samples for a statistically valid study of the CSF of hypomagnesaemic cows. But he did help me with a larger study of serum magnesium levels.

Some of the call-outs were quite dramatic. Grass staggers was more of a problem in some herds than others. Even some of the supposedly "normal" cows in these herds seemed to be particularly touchy. A critical time was when they came in for milking. A farmer would start putting the cups onto a tense and excitable cow. She would lash out with a foot. He would swear at her. The tension in the shed was raised a notch, and she would fall over and start convulsing. Sometimes, in her aimless thrashings, she might drag herself under the bars and tip into the milking pit, totally disrupting the milking session. Tension is transmissible between cows and men, and all hell could break loose as other hypomagnesaemic cows caught the mood. The farmer might end up with a couple of cows upside down flailing their legs in the pit and a couple of others thrashing about on the platform. Pandemonium reigns. Call the vet!

We blood tested the supposedly normal cows on these farms to find out why they were so susceptible to grass staggers. Quite often the results came back within the expected reference range for serum magnesium, a bit on the low side, perhaps, but taken in isolation each cow could be said to be "normal". However, we noticed that the reference ranges used by the animal health laboratories in New Zealand were considerably lower than those I had been familiar with in Britain. When we found that our samples from several herds were consistently on the low side of "normal" we wondered whether the data used in NZ cows was skewed because New Zealand cows were chronically deficient in magnesium, and if so why? John, Hank and I also had a hunch that hypomagnesaemia was more prevalent in herds using high levels of potash fertilizer. It was known that potassium competes with magnesium for uptake by pasture, so these animals were probably grazing grass low in magnesium. This was difficult to prove directly because the magnesium levels in pasture fluctuate rapidly from day to day. As I went round the herds taking blood samples, it also became apparent that chronic hypomagnesaemia was tied in with other conditions such as "Taranaki anaemia" and an udder affliction the local farmers called "leatherbag" (also "caked udder" or "rubber bag"). To my regret when we published an article about this in the *New Zealand Veterinary Journal* we were advised to use a more scientific name, so we coined the rather unimaginative term "chronic udder oedema". These cows had a persistent thick swelling at the base of their udders which, once it had formed, would never go away and could be bad enough to interfere with their ability to release milk. The thickening tended to worsen with each season, and leatherbag cows usually had to be culled prematurely.

Our paper seemed to trigger some interest. The reference ranges the animal health laboratories recommended for serum magnesium levels in cattle were raised, and some veterinary scientists descended on us with blood tubes and sample pottles and co-opted me to take them onto the worst affected farms. The pottles were for urine. There was a new test to measure the concentrations of magnesium in urine. It's easy enough to suck the blood out of the tail vein of a cow, but how do you make a cow urinate on demand? Once again, the doctors have it over us vets…

It requires some patience, but if you rhythmically rub the skin beneath a cow's vulva she will generally oblige. It's not the sort of thing you want to be found doing without good reason. It could be quite time-consuming and there was always the odd cow that wouldn't release. Invariably we were the butt of ribald comments; farmers never let vets off the hook if they can help it: "If you carry on like that she'll be doing you for harassment!" Sometimes you had to give up, or try again later and sometimes there were accidents … There I was, stroking away, my mind on some higher plane, when a cow lifted her tail and filled my gumboots… but not with urine. The old farmer gave me a wry smile: "Must have pressed the wrong button there, son."

By this stage many farmers were finding that if they supplemented their cows with magnesium during spring, their cows were generally less nervy, easier to milk and gave more milk. They also had fewer occurrences of full-blown grass staggers. Over the next few years most New Zealand dairy farmers adopted this practice and, these days, not only are there some very sophisticated automated systems for delivering magnesium supplements to dairy cows, but there is also a far greater understanding of the interactions between minerals in the soil and pasture and the need to be cautious about the timing and rates of application of all fertilizers, but especially potash.

I like to think that John Pauli and I contributed a small amount to the understanding of a topic which had such important implications for New Zealand's dairy industry; for, as *Blood and Henderson* stated: "Tetany associated with depression of serum magnesium levels is a common occurrence in ruminants, but probably in no other disease of domestic animals is there as much confusion in relation to aetiology and pathogenesis as there is in this group of diseases. The position is made even more confusing by the variety of circumstances in which they occur, and by their common association with other metabolic and nutritional deficiency diseases."

My rewarding early experience of trial work encouraged me into further scientific trials on farms later in my career. I especially enjoyed working alongside farmers who were willing, often at considerable inconvenience and cost to themselves, to provide their animals and give their time for the greater good and the cause of science. Many of our investigations revealed the worthlessness of supplements peddled unethically to farmers for whom the real answers usually lay in improved management and better nutrition. Apart from the provision of essential trace elements, where they are known to be deficient, and controlling internal parasites, the three most important things contributing to healthy and productive livestock remain—as we were so strongly advised as students—*feeding, feeding and feeding*.

~

My copy of *Blood and Henderson* was inscribed by my fiancée: Darling John, for our engagement... with all my love, Viv. That was the start of her lifelong commitment to my career, as was the case for so many vets' wives of that and previous generations. My *Blood and Henderson* was a brand new and expensive 1968 edition; cheaper second-hand copies had not yet found their way into the student bookshops. To some it would seem an unromantic gift, but Viv had invested her hard-earned money in my future, in my passion to be a vet. No present could have thrilled me more.

It is strange how the passions that drive us change. Many people retain their passions for their careers, sometimes at the expense of that for their partners. For me it was the other way round. Failed marriages are a hazard for vets as much as anyone else, but the current growing disaffection of vets for their profession is not talked about, nor expected by the general public, who are still mislead by Herriotism. This is a term coined by modern vets to describe the legacy left by the brilliant novels of James Herriot and his romanticised depiction of veterinary practice in the 1930s. Some aspects of Herriotism survive in modern veterinary practice, but social changes have ensured his model of life as a vet has all but vanished. One of the reasons why so many young vets are abandoning their profession early is that the idealised perceptions they harbour as young undergraduates do not match up with the reality they now find behind the farm gate.

I have to confess that I embraced the James Herriot myth for all it was worth. I feel lucky that I was born in an era where I could be that sort of vet—well, some of the time. For the most part of my working life I couldn't imagine doing anything else or, perhaps more importantly, being anything else. Being a vet was my identity.

But, against the immense satisfaction vetting generally brought me, there were certainly some doubts and darker moments.

Chapter Twenty-five

The Seeds of Doubt

The bond between a man and his profession is similar to that which ties him to his country; it is just as complex, often ambivalent, and in general it is understood completely only when it is broken: by exile or emigration in the case of one's country, by retirement in the case of a trade or profession. – Primo Levi

I looked at the handwritten envelope in front of me. I didn't recognise the writing. It was early January: a delayed Christmas card? Well, not exactly. It read "I hope you have a lousy New Year". An attached letter explained that the dog I had recently treated had since died, "thanks to you". It was signed "yours hatefully, Buddy". (Not his real name.)

I only had to think back a few days to recall Buddy. I had been called out on Christmas Day to see his Boxer dog, Fritz, who had suffered a sudden bout of vomiting and diarrhoea after eating some fish bait. When I examined him, Fritz had been a bit subdued, as could be expected, and I had treated him for a routine gastro-enteritis, a diagnosis consistent with the history and presenting signs. I always made it a policy not to assume that my patients would automatically recover from my treatments, so I did warn Buddy to get in touch if Fritz didn't get better or, more importantly, if he deteriorated.

Buddy, a fisherman, had been thrilled that I could see him at such short notice. Both he and I were unable to contact his usual vet. After I had attended to Fritz he had even talked about dropping off some crayfish for me and we parted on warm terms.

Until I received this entirely unexpected and obnoxious card I had obviously been deluded in my assumption that Fritz had made an uneventful recovery. Whereas—the letter continued—when Fritz collapsed the next day Buddy had... taken him straight round to his usual vet [the one he was unable to contact on Christmas Day], who told him that Fritz had kidney failure and that if only he had seen Fritz earlier he would have been able to save him. How could he be so sure?

Apart from the upset of Fritz's death I felt betrayed by the other vet. He could have had only the vaguest idea of what I had done for Fritz. His throwaway comment may have been purely to promote his own abilities but he was, by implication, denigrating mine. Was he also aware that he had sown hatred in the mind of Fritz's owner? As a registered vet he should have been aware of his ethical obligations and known that the correct procedure should have been to contact me and find out more about my diagnosis and treatment so that he could tailor his more effectively. It was a blatant case of "supersession".

The internal workings of the professions are subject to great suspicion by those who regard them as stuffy, protectionist and anti-competitive, but they would be re-assured if they read the Code of Professional Conduct to which vets are supposed to adhere. It is largely concerned with maintaining standards of care and competence:

Veterinarians must take into consideration the risks of treating an animal without first ascertaining from the original veterinarian the initial diagnosis and details of any treatment prescribed. Making such enquiries will normally safeguard the interests of the animal, the legal position of the veterinarians concerned and enable the professional courtesies implicit in this rule to be observed.

If it is discovered during the course of a consultation that the patient has been in the care of another veterinarian for the same reason, then the latter should be notified as soon as possible after the consultation. The welfare of the animal must be the overriding consideration under all circumstances.

The unfairness of Buddy's accusation certainly upset me and it did result in repercussions for his vet. It wasn't the first time he had trodden on our toes. I had good records of my clinical work-up for Fritz, and I forwarded them plus my "greetings" card to the New Zealand Veterinary Council. I felt vindicated when the vet concerned was censured for his unethical behaviour.

Ever since the Veterinary Surgeons Act of 1881, veterinary surgeons could, theoretically, be removed from the Register for "disgraceful professional conduct", but to begin with, the Council of the Royal College of Veterinary Surgeons could not decide what constituted such an offence. They initially jumped on advertising, always a contentious issue for vets.

Even as early as 1890 there was acute competition between veterinarians. Times were hard and vets were distributing circulars offering cut-price services. The Council then received a complaint about one member who was promoting his services and "nostrums" by blowing a hunting horn in the local marketplace. It may sound colourful and quaint to our ears, but this was regarded as a flagrant case of unprofessional advertising and in 1894 advertising became the first item listed as "conduct disgraceful in a professional respect".

These days the Commerce Commission would almost certainly protect the rights of the horn blower against any edicts from his profession, but this reflects a relatively recent change of opinion. For much of my career advertising was strictly proscribed. It was felt preferable that your abilities be promoted by word of mouth. Most vets were reasonably happy with that, because it freed them to concentrate on providing a good service rather than waste their energy blowing horns. But there has always been the counter argument that the profession needed to lift its profile, promote itself, and inform the public about the wide range of services it offers. Over recent years, veterinary practices have grown bigger and their staff less stable; their clientele is also more mobile, displays less loyalty and shops around for the best deals. If you want to compete you have to advertise. Vets who find the new ethos personally distasteful can always employ others to run their promotions. We have reached the stage where many practices employ CEOs and run advertising budgets. So the Code has been modified and advertising is now sanctioned, a cause lost or won, depending on your point of view; but there are many other pitfalls in the Code for the maverick vet.

Most veterinarians employed in western countries will glance, gloat or shudder through the reviews published by their respective disciplinary bodies. There, paraded as a warning for all to heed, are the misdeeds of those miscreants who have, in the opinion of their peers, stepped over the boundaries. This could be for a variety of offences: drug addiction, supplying false certification, professional negligence or straight incompetence. The worst transgressors are "struck off" the Register—their means of livelihood removed for varying periods of time.

I felt the most sympathy for a British vet who was severely censured by the Royal College of Veterinary Surgeons for killing a hamster. He picked the unfortunate animal from its cage and—I can imagine his instinctive reaction when the little creature bit him on the thumb—flicked it off, unfortunately killing it in the process. It must have been the way he performed this "highly unprofessional" manoeuvre that resulted in the owner laying a complaint. I can almost hear the profanity exploding from his lips. So many disciplinary cases proceed through lack of communication or empathy. A heartfelt apology by the "hamster thug" at the time may have prevented a lot of anguish and expense, but maybe he was unlucky enough to strike a particularly obdurate owner. I can't recall if he took up his right of appeal to the Privy Council but, if he had, it would have ended up as an extremely expensive hamster.

The dispensing and sale of dangerous or restricted drugs is another contentious area. What does an assertive farmer or horse owner care for professional ethics? There will always be those who attempt to browbeat vets into supplying inappropriate antibiotics for food producing animals, or anabolic steroids to make a winning horse out of a loser. The vet who takes a firm ethical stand risks condemnation for being officious and losing business for his employer. The lax vet gains friends and attracts business at the risk of alienating his colleagues and facing disciplinary action. Vets' obligations to the national interest—in matters such as biosecurity, the prevention of drug residues in animal products and to police animal welfare infractions—override any obligation to keep a client happy. Striking a balance between ethics and pragmatism was never easy, but it has become increasingly stressful: especially for young vets at the start of their careers.

~

As nasty letters go, Buddy's lacked subtlety. One of the most unpleasant letters I ever received was as a university student from the Dean of the Veterinary Faculty. I was never a brilliant student, but I was diligent. I worked very hard throughout my years of study. At the end of my fourth year I was relieved to have passed all my exams. Viv and I had been married for one year, and after I had worked through most of the summer vacation with a local vet, we decided to recharge our batteries and go on a walking holiday on the Isle of Mull. There we learned that camping in late summer amongst the midges in the Scottish Highlands is an experience to be avoided at all costs. New Zealand sandflies are positively benign by comparison. On the way home, tired and happy, I ran our car into the back of a long queue of vehicles. They were unexpectedly parked round a bend in the road beside the traffic-jammed banks of Loch Lomond. I set up a chain of nose to tail crashes. Inconvenient insurance claims ensued. When we finally arrived home to our flat we attacked the pile of mail awaiting us. There was a neatly typed letter from the Dean's office:

Dear Mr Hicks,
I write to inform you that although you passed in the recent B.V.Sc. examination in Pharmacology this was only a marginal pass. You should attempt to achieve a higher standard of performance in future examinations.
Yours sincerely etc.

I had long forgotten this incident, but it recently came to light—the words preserved in a letter Viv had written to her mother. She'd added "John took it very much to heart" and that she'd torn it up, observing to her mother that I was the last person to need that sort of "encouragement". Viv salved some of my hurt by pointing out that "Mr Hicks" and "Pharmacology" were filled in on a standard letterform, so I was not the sole recipient of this letter of admonishment. What was most surprising was that hitherto the Prof. had been a distant academic who had little or no contact with his students. He would no more have been able to put a face to my name than I were the Chinese artisan who carved the ivory tower from which he was pontificating. His letter had reduced me to my childhood, the school reports in which the master writes "could try harder" or "must learn to be less careless": comments from loose canons which were sometimes perceptive, but frequently well wide of the mark.

University days are claimed by many to be the happiest of their lives, but for me they were more or less a continuation of school. Since those all-important 'O' levels, which had set me on the path to becoming a vet, I had endured eight years of exams. With finals approaching I had one to go. I couldn't wait to escape academia and start to earn my living as a "proper" vet. It was the practical stuff that filled my dreams—and those of most of my year mates. Not for us life behind a desk nor, even, a laboratory bench. It seemed a strange waste of a veterinary degree to pursue such goals; yet that, increasingly, seems to be where many of today's veterinary graduates end up, if they stay in the profession at all, for they have been selected on academic ability alone.

While I had struggled with the drier academic subjects in my veterinary course I revelled in the practical work and loved accompanying vets on their rounds. And when I qualified I rejoiced in the sheer variety of my work: the satisfaction of seeing the interlocking fragments of a jagged fracture drawn together by a well placed compression plate, the relief of finally flicking the head of a calf round so that it was aligned and ready to be delivered, the drama of toppling a large horse under anaesthesia. It's hardly "raindrops on roses" or "warm woollen mittens" stuff, especially when you've been targeted by a nasty hind and the raindrops are a maelstrom of blows raining on your head; or you face the agony of a thousand cows lined up for pregnancy testing and the warm woollen mittens defy description. But why would the Prof. want to trade all that for life behind a Bunsen burner? Perhaps he didn't apply himself sufficiently during his clinical years.

Fortunately for me, that last year of the veterinary course was particularly interesting, and I can still vividly recall some of our more entertaining days in the field. Perhaps the Prof. had done me a favour. Mental vigour is required of the practising vet: acceptance and rebuttal, success and failure will be recurring themes throughout his working life. We win some, we lose some.

Chapter Twenty-six

Win Some, Lose Some

Success is the ability to go from failure to failure without losing your enthusiasm. – Winston Churchill

Don and Jane were unusual immigrants. Don was a chirpy cockney, an irrepressible extrovert, the life and soul of any party. Although a born and bred city lad, his dream was to farm. In those days (1960s) most immigrants travelled to New Zealand by boat. On the long trip from England Don met Jane, a Scottish lass who shared his dream. Shortly after disembarking in Wellington, they were married. They worked on dairy farms, gaining experience. When we first knew them in Taranaki they were sharemilkers with a young family, starting to work up the ladder of increasing ownership until they could build up a herd of their own and, eventually, buy their own farm. For aspiring farmers, New Zealand was a land of opportunity.

Apart from the odd farm visit, I met Don regularly at net practices and for Saturday afternoon cricket. He was the captain of a motley team comprising freezing workers, stock agents, a banker, several dairy farmers and Neil, an older man—purportedly the author of steamy novels. It was new territory for me, a joshing world of nicknames: of Maoris called "Albi" and red-haired Celts called "Blue". Don was a born leader: perennially cheerful, a natural wit, master of repartee and a fair-minded sportsman, always offering encouragement to the younger players, never holding back on affectionate sarcasm for the slow and lumbering older members of his team. This was third grade stuff but, what we lacked in talent, we made up for in enthusiasm. There was no slackness in our team; we were keen, we played hard and we had fun. These were the same values Don and Jane applied to their working life. Viv and I became part of their circle of friends.

One evening Don phoned me urgently. "John, I've got a very sick calf."

I made a half-hearted protest. "Don, I'm not on duty. Have you tried the after-hours…?"

"I'm sorry John, but this is something special, and I'd prefer a friend to deal with it."

He'd pressed the right buttons. We all like to be needed by those we love and respect. What else could I do but drop what I was doing and rush out to the farm?

As we walked to the calf shed he filled me in on the details. "Sorry to drag you out John, but this is a very special calf."

"We really liked the look of Red Polls when we went back home," he continued, referring to a recent visit he and Jane had made to Britain to catch up with their relatives. Red Polls are a rare breed of English cattle. "The closest we could get to them here was Danish Red. So we inseminated six of our Shorthorns with Danish Red semen this year. Unfortunately we only got one heifer calf, a beautiful wee thing and— beggar me—she would be the one with the scours this morning."

"Did you give her any treatment, Don?"

"I thought it was just a case of white scours. I gave her a sulpha tablet, but she was lying in a heap when I went to feed them tonight—just before I rang you. I think she's a hopeless case, but we want to give her every chance."

Paradoxically, most vets enjoy getting their hands on what an owner considers to be a "hopeless case". You are off the hook if your patient dies, but there is always the slight chance of pulling off a miracle and becoming a hero. But when I saw that calf lying motionless and sunken-eyed—deeply dehydrated—I, too, felt that this was a hopeless case.

"Throw the book at her John. She could be the founding member of our new herd."

As a student I'd had the great fortune to see practice with George Rafferty, a vet in the Highlands of Scotland who was an advocate of blood transfusions for collapsed calves. He had developed a practical method for farm use—one that would make a human physician cringe—but farm animal practice is ever the art of compromise. For a start, he'd cut out cross-matching of donor and recipient blood beforehand. In cattle, as in dogs, reactions to a first transfusion are rare and, unlike human medicine, the chance of a calf receiving a second one in its lifetime is extremely remote.

Apart from restoring a collapsed circulation, transfused cow's blood contains important antibodies against the diseases present on the farm. Given intravenously, these are mainlined directly into the calf's system where they can act immediately. How many more people and animals would have survived through history if doctors and vets had mastered the secrets of transfusing blood into the body; as against all the harm they inflicted by blood letting out of it?

First, we needed a compliant cow. Don walked one of the quietest members of his herd into the milking shed and, without her consent—as is the habit of vets—I tightened a cord round her neck to raise a jugular vein and, when it was obvious, injected some local anaesthetic over it. I then made a short cut along her jugular with a scalpel and rotated the blade against the flow. A bright stream of blood splashed into my flask and I rocked it steadily, mixing it with some sodium citrate anticoagulant. It was critical that there were no clots. It was not long before our gentle donor, minus a few pints of blood and with a couple of stitches in her neck, was freed back into her paddock—perhaps to ruminate on the strangeness of mankind.

Our patient, by contrast, seemed past caring. I was quite unable to locate her jugular vein, shrivelled as it was, beneath the tacky skin of her neck. She was in a state of circulatory collapse. I had to resort to cutting through the skin and dissecting down onto the thin blue streak her jugular had become. I eased a cannula into it and connected it to my flask of blood using the rubber tubing and a flutter valve I normally used for calcium solutions to treat cows with milk fever. But blood is thicker than calcium borogluconate; how very slowly that blood trickled in! It was easy to see why most busy practitioners, rushing around attending all those urgent calls in spring, had not adopted George Rafferty's technique.

Don was tiring of his job of holding up the flask. He fetched a pitchfork and propped it against the wall. We hung the flask off one of the tines. It formed an effective, if rustic, drip-stand. We concentrated on our patient, looking for any signs of improvement, willing her to respond. We propped her up with armfuls of straw. In that crude, dimly lit calf shed a scene of almost biblical intensity was unfolding. But, as the minutes ticked by, a miracle seemed less and less likely. Our calf lay still and, save for its feeble, irregular heart beat, to all intents and purposes, lifeless. We left the pen with half the blood still to run— abandoning our patient to her fate. A wee dram was

233

called for, and we hadn't the heart to check up on her when I left for home.

The phone rang early the next morning. Don sounded perhaps more perky than usual, but it wasn't his style to let on straight away. He started with the weather. "Oh! Don," I interrupted, "If you're passing the clinic sometime today, could you drop off…?" I was going to ask for the gear I'd left behind in the calf shed.

"Hold on, hold on, you little beauty! You'll never guess what's happened to Viv."

"Viv?"

"Yes, that's what we're calling the calf."

"The one we treated last night?"

"The very one. She was up and nuzzling my hand for a feed this morning! We couldn't call her John. Anyway, it would probably go to your head, like the five wickets you took against Kaponga last summer. So we've named her in honour of your dear wife!"

Poor Viv: she turned out to be an unproductive beast, and was culled a couple of years later. Farming is a business. Sentiment on a farm can only run so far. Danish Reds never caught on in New Zealand. A shame, really. There are few prettier sights than red cattle set against lush, green pasture. But this happy story is, in my mind, inextricably linked to a far darker and more puzzling one.

When we left the district, we kept in touch with Don and Jane. Christmas letters told us of their progress. They had at last realised their dream and bought their own farm. A daughter was married. Don was branching into another business utilising his public speaking and motivational skills. Then the letters stopped. From an old colleague we learned that Don was dead. He'd been found by one of his children, hanging, in a shed. We, as the many other friends who loved his seemingly unquenchable spirit, cannot answer the sad questions that recur whenever we think of him.

~

In some ways you could say that Big Dave is like Don, a cheerful, booming presence. He could easily have stepped, black-vested, out of a Barry Crump novel. A visit to his farm would, to misquote that favourite piece of parental advice, almost certainly end in laughter. But when he rang me early one morning, it sounded serious.

Dave is one of a line of horsemen: men who have horses in their blood and love their power, danger and mystery. In the 1980s quite a few Southland sheep farmers had a loose box or two, kept a few mares, and bred and raced trotters, pacers or gallopers. Their numbers have dwindled as sheep farming has become less profitable and farmers busier, with less leisure time to indulge an expensive and time-consuming hobby. While Dave was always great company, with a laugh-a-minute sense of humour, I knew he had a healthy disdain for politicians and, I fancied, a detached sense of irony towards the veterinary profession. In his eyes, I imagined, we really were no better, nor worse than any of the other parasites clamouring for farmers' hard earned dollars. He certainly sounded as though he held no great expectations when he rang me about his valuable foal just as I was about to drive to work:

"I wouldn't have interrupted your beauty sleep if I felt I could have done something myself", was his first salvo. "But this is a really valuable foal." He strung off the name of the mother's sire and dam, as horse people do. It could have been by Smegma out of Borborygmi, but it meant nothing to me, I have never followed the racing game. However, in those days we did see quite a few horses and I hoped I would be able to do something to raise Dave's opinion of my noble calling. If he had set me a challenge he thought I was unequal to, I would show him!

As I turned into the drive, I paused to wave as Wendy, his wife, pulled out on her way to work. I parked in the yard. The paint on the rotten weatherboards of the cold, dingy, farmhouse in which Dave and Wendy had raised their family was peeling into lank grass. Across the way, a brand new edifice had taken its place. Wendy's protests had born fruit. She had finally cajoled Dave into making their living accommodation a priority over his beloved horses. The new kitset home they had lovingly assembled, despite months of frustrating delays and setbacks, was her pride and joy.

It was a bitterly cold morning. The young foal lying in the mud at her mother's feet was virtually comatose. Occasionally, a feeble spasm wracked her body. There was no helpful history. According to Dave she had been up and suckling last night. Mum, standing patiently by her sick foal, seemed fretful, but was otherwise fine. I checked her milk—there was plenty, so she hadn't been suckled for a while. Perhaps the foal had succumbed to neonatal maladjustment syndrome, NMS, where foals, brain damaged at birth, suddenly become "barkers", "dummies" or "wanderers". With careful nursing they often recover. But our foal was cold, barely conscious and close to death. It seemed hopeless. If only Dave had lain in bed an extra hour! Sometimes it is a relief for a vet to arrive just after the patient has died. How much easier it is not to have to toss up whether to "give it a go" or declare the case "hopeless". This time "hopeless" was realistic, but "hopeless" wouldn't do. My patient still clung to life, however tenuously, and she was only of any value to Dave if she lived to race.

I needed thinking time. I resorted to the old thermometer trick. It would be interesting to see just how cold she was.

A minute passed and, even though I had shaken the thermometer right down before inserting it, it had not risen one iota. I hadn't expected it to. Neither, I could see from the doubting look on his face, had Dave. But I had hatched a plan. "Look Dave, I'm sorry, but the foal is severely hypothermic. She's dying of exposure. There must be an underlying reason for her collapse, but the first thing we're going to have to do is try and raise her body temperature."

"How do you intend to do that?"

"Well…" I should have paused for longer, he who hesitates is sometimes very sensible; but an optimistic vision of success—of showing Dave just how wise he was to call on my services—flashed through my mind. "Look Dave, they are now treating hypothermia cases in people by total immersion in hot water. If we can raise her core temperature to something like normal, we might then stand a chance of finding out more about the underlying problem. We'll just have to tackle it one step at a time."

As soon as the words left my mouth I realised I was committing myself to a time-consuming and probably futile intervention; a move I would likely regret. But I had offered hope. It was too late to retract, so I modified my confident pronouncement with a touch of realism. "It really is a long shot."

"We need to get the foal into a bath of hot water." I continued. I was thinking about a discarded bath, perhaps one now used as a water trough, or what about the old house? But the power was off, the fittings gutted. By a process of elimination, I managed to extract the inevitable from Dave's very own lips: a bath with lashings of hot water was only available in the new house. We'd have to use the new house.

"You don't know what you're asking, John. Wendy will kill me if she finds out." It seemed strange coming from Big Dave, looming well over six feet in his stockinged feet, but before long he had entered into the spirit of the occasion. We kicked off our boots at the front door, a token concession to matrimonial harmony. The clean fresh paint and wallpaper was assailed by the smell of honest sweat and horse manure. We hefted our patient—heavy, mud-slimed and slippery—towards the bathroom. Precariously, we paused to re-grip, staggered our way across the light and airy living area, threaded past a cream lounge suite, and round a few tight corners down a narrow hall. With our hands fully occupied it was impossible to prevent the aimless, convulsive paddling of dirt-laden hooves. A trail of mud peppered the oatmeal carpet. Occasional dollops disappeared onto the walls—disguising themselves amongst the rose-strewn wallpaper, awaiting chance discovery on some happy occasion in the future. Dave, the last person I would have taken as house proud, tried to keep track of these, but he was a man distracted. Soon we were both carried away by the surreal absurdity of the situation. "It's all right for you. You'll be able to bugger off in a couple of hours when you've killed my foal. I'll be welded to a vacuum cleaner for the rest of the day."

"Aw, get away with you! It will be a bit more cottagey with some genuine horse shit on the walls," I ventured.

"Go on! Joke about it! You won't be here when Wendy comes back." His jocular tone failed to disguise an element of fear. I made a mental note to make sure I wouldn't be.

The bathroom was tastefully decorated—clean and bright; but I had no time to admire the subtle, pastel shades. There was a logistical problem to solve.

Archimedes, wise Greek that he was, must have filled his bath prior to getting into it. This option was not open to us, we had to deposit our burden first. With some relief, we slithered our filthy foal into the pristine white bath. Freed at last, my soiled daubs were soon defiling the gleaming gold mixer tap, and we filled the bath around her.

At this point, it is pertinent to note that baths designed for the human body are not the right shape to accommodate a foal. We achieved a reasonable fit with the foal laid on its back. Instinctively, she rejected this unnatural position, even in her semi-comatose state. As the water level rose she became more difficult to restrain. Her long limbs, still absently paddling away, refused to fold neatly into place. As I concentrated on supporting her head above water it was becoming increasingly obvious that there were problems at the other end. Big Dave may have been as strong as an ox, but he was proving to be considerably less adroit than an octopus. Liberal sprays of hot, muddy water flicked across plush towelling, dribbled down the delicate dado and strobed across the complicated clutter of shampoos and cosmetics on glass shelves. That gave me an idea.

"Perhaps we could tidy up with some of Wendy's ex*fol*iating lotion."

My feeble effort was peremptorily dismissed: "I'm more worried about excommunication if Wendy finds

239

out!" "If" seemed an increasingly optimistic qualification, given the circumstances.

Sometime, during our struggles, there came a "eureka!" moment of near perfect immersion. By some chance of timing we had achieved an almost complete displacement of water. A tide of filth ran along the floor. Archimedes would have been proud of us, but perhaps he didn't have carpet in the hallway next to his bathroom…

Mercifully, it took far less than two hours for the foal to expire. One final flurry of flaying limbs, and she was dead. The clean up job promised to take a lot longer.

Dave seemed to take his loss philosophically, but now the charade had played its course, the time for jokes was past. I helped him carry the body outside. My quick post-mortem was inconclusive. I needed to extract the brain for laboratory tests if I was to find the cause, but Dave, realistically, declined the further expense. Besides, he seemed desperate to get on with the housework. For a fraction of a second I pictured his tall, lean figure in a black-vested frenzy of muscular mopping, driving a damp duster round the Crown Derby, or sponging horse shit off the chintz. Perhaps the wry smile I tried to suppress, as he waved me away, would be my undoing. I scurried back to my car, consigning Dave's fate to his dubious skills as a house husband.

A day or two later I was surprised and relieved to hear, from the safety of my desk at the back of our clinic, a cheery voice and noisy laughter rattling the walls of the reception area. Dave sounded his usual, vital self. Wendy must have enjoyed an inordinately happy day at work, the day we messed her house up. Or Dave must have resorted to low cunning. A strategic meal out? A bunch of roses? It didn't seem his style. I listened as he spoke to one of the girls. Was there an edge to his booming request? Perhaps something more than detached irony? "Now, where's that Hicks fellow? Tell him I want to see him now."

It was time to hide.

~

The story of the foal in the bath is a somewhat rueful footnote to my involvement with horses. To set the record straight, Dave is not the sort of person to hold a grudge. I am pleased to report that we were on friendly terms when we last met socially.

Horses have challenged and pained me totally out of proportion to other species during my veterinary career. In this respect horses *are* different. They cost a lot to buy and to keep. They are large, strong and can be dangerous. The faster and more valuable they are, the more they live on a physiological knife-edge. They and their owners present the greatest challenge to vets, an observation backed up by the disproportionately large number of professional indemnity insurance claims made by horse owners against vets each year. Horse vets are unwise if they don't take out additional insurance cover. Death and disaster are never far away.

One common procedure, as much as any other in his repertoire, highlights the drama of a horse vet's life: general anaesthesia. Horse anaesthesia is always a challenge. Guinea-pig anaesthesia has its attendant risks, but it is equine anaesthesia I am drawn to write about …

Chapter Twenty-seven

The Sleep of Life

Below the thunders of the upper deep;
Far, far beneath in the abysmal sea,
His ancient, dreamless, uninvaded sleep
The Kraken sleepeth.
- Alfred, Lord Tennyson

By a quirk of human nature we are always impressed by the latest whizz-bang technology, even if it isn't the best. It has been claimed that for reliability, rate of fire and overall effectiveness, English longbows, as used at the famous English victory at Agincourt in 1415, were not surpassed by muskets for three hundred years and, in the hands of trained archers, they could still have been effective tactical weapons at the battle of Waterloo four hundred years later. Yet the military, impressed by noise and technology fell, erringly, for the more unreliable musket. It seems that the development of veterinary anaesthetics has sometimes followed a similar path.

Horses can be awkward animals to anaesthetise. One of the commonest reasons to, in veterinary slang, "knock a horse down" is for the routine operation of castration, though perhaps there is more poetry in the older word: *geld*. Gelding a horse can be quite a challenge for the vet concerned, since it usually precedes the painstaking process of breaking a horse in—the process that makes horses tractable to the whim of men and wiles of women. Unbroken colts can be decidedly frisky and untrustworthy.

242

As vet students, before we qualified, we had one memorable bus trip to a farm in Derbyshire. Awaiting our arrival were about twenty semi-wild ponies. They had been mustered off the moors and corralled into a large stone-walled field. Our task was to castrate them and compare several different anaesthetic techniques. The traditional method involved strapping a canvas nosebag (a Cox's mask) onto the muzzle and then inserting a chloroform soaked sponge through a zippered compartment, close to the nostrils. Another group of horses were knocked out with a dose of barbiturate. This is a very reliable, but highly irritant chemical, and it must be injected into a vein—the jugular in the neck being the most accessible. It is essential not to inject any barbiturate around the vein, which is easier said than done with a prancing horse; any mistake and there is likely to be a severe reaction followed, in a day or two, by sepsis (pus formation). An abscess around the jugular can be fatal. The last method we tested that day was the newly available drug "Immobilon", a version of the drug used to dart African game animals. It had the great advantage that a vein was not required; it could be injected into a muscle. A large muscle mass, such as in the side of the neck, is a much easier target than a vein.

The traditional tried and trusted chloroform worked very well. These ponies were walked slowly round in a big circle and soon relaxed and slid to the ground as the drug took effect. The Immobilon worked, but the ponies seemed stressed under its influence. They were tense, and shook and trembled—sometimes making the operation difficult to perform. Fortunately there was an antagonist, "Revivon", which quickly reversed the Immobilon and the ponies were on their feet in a jiffy. The Immobilon/Revivon combination gave by far the quickest recovery time, a definite advantage not only for the horse, but also the vet who has to wait around to supervise the risky recovery period when a half-doped horse can run into fences or other obstacles and injure itself. The barbiturate was all right as long as the pony was under control at the time of the injection. The vein had to be punctured competently first time; our ponies, much as their human counterparts would be, were reluctant about repeated stabbings. Unfortunately, there is no effective reversal agent for barbiturate anaesthesia and the ponies injected with it took a long time to recover and needed careful supervision while they came round.

To the casual observer, chloroform would have appeared the best option. Unfortunately, its use was becoming unacceptable. Vets were becoming aware of its toxicity to the liver and the fatal risk this carried, especially if the horse was not a fit young animal.

Each method had its drawbacks. By the time I started working in New Zealand a couple of years later, the use of chloroform was proscribed and Immobilon was not available for the very good reason that it was a risky drug for the humans using it. A small dose could prove fatal and the risk of accidental self-injection while dealing with a bouncy horse was too great. Purposeful self-injection was another matter. There had been several Immobilon suicides by vets and vet nurses in Britain, where the drug was readily available.

There was a further option for the brave horse vet. This was standing castration: sneaking up boldly—a valid paradox when considering a puny human weighing perhaps one tenth of the half-tonne kicking machine he was setting himself against—and using local anaesthetic alone. Gliding a needle through the tender scrotal skin without the horse objecting is not easy.

In New Zealand the most commonly used general anaesthetic technique was to inject a barbiturate drug, such as thiopentone, directly into the jugular vein.

So it was that one fine Canterbury morning my friend Kit asked me to accompany him to geld a Clydesdale. Clydesdales were once the commonest work horses on New Zealand farms. A few remain, mostly in the hands of hobbyists. Normally gelding is a job for one vet but, with such a large and valuable animal, it seemed better for two of us to attend. Even though he was only a yearling, he towered above us. Fortunately, he was a pleasure to work with: placid-natured—as are most animals bred for work rather than for sport.

Everyone was relaxed as we injected the sedative. While this was working we prepared our instruments and equipment—rope, cotton wool, scalpel, triple crush emasculators, tetanus antiserum, penicillin injection, and antiseptic powder. We dissolved a couple of five gram bottles of thiopentone, each in fifty millilitres of sterile water and injected a bleb of local into the skin over the colt's jugular vein with a fine needle. He never flinched. The worst part was done … he shouldn't feel the wide bore needle, through which we planned to carefully inject the large volume of thio necessary to drop him.

Confident we had everything under control we instructed the owner what to expect next. "It will take eight to ten seconds after Kit has injected him for the drug to take effect. That's when you'll have to concentrate, because he'll pull back hard." We prepared for this and, given the size of our patient, two men were put on the rope attached to his head collar. I was one of them. "There's always a danger that he'll pull so hard that he'll topple over backwards and bang his head. We must keep the tension on the rope and try to keep his head off the ground until he has relaxed into the anaesthetic." We eased the colt into an open position. All was clear behind him.

Kit inserted a large eighteen-gauge needle into the jugular. The dark red splash on his hand indicated a clean strike. Deftly, he connected the first syringe and emptied it, discarded it, and repeated with the next one. "Fifty mils, John. Anytime now!" We braced ourselves, facing the colt. Seconds passed. Suddenly the colt reared on his hind legs, front feet waving way, way above our heads. We were jerked off our feet. For all the tension we could put on that rope we may as well have been lice on a strand of hair.

What the f***!

We scattered as, unexpectedly, he ran forwards, did a complete somersault and came to rest twenty metres behind us, under a hedge. He lay there relaxed, breathing deeply and appeared to be unharmed. More to the point, so were we. It took a while for four of us to drag him into a more convenient place for his operation, which proceeded without any further hitches. It was a salutary lesson for two young vets: learn to anticipate the unexpected.

Sometime later I saw a master demonstrate yet another approach to dealing with horse castrations. Gordon Burr sedated his horses, just as we had; but then he resorted to ropes: a combination of new and old technologies. He placed a thick leather collar round the horse's neck, and hobbles round the fetlocks (ankles) of each hind foot. He drew up one hind leg and tied it to the collar. Then, as the horse was pushed back, the rope on the other back leg was shortened. The horse, quite naturally, sank to the ground, and lay on its side. The second hind leg was also trussed tightly to the collar. It was like watching a ballet—a combination of timing and balance. With unhurried grace all four legs were neatly folded and roped. Gordon's horses hardly fought; they knew they were helpless. In a matter of moments they were parcelled as neatly as a fly by a spider. It was then a simple matter for him to inject the local anaesthetic around the scrotum and conduct the surgery safely and humanely. Of all the techniques I have seen this was the most impressive. It was safe for horse and operator, used a minimum of drugs, and was entirely humane. However, it required a certain physicality and consummate skill on the part of the operator. Gordon was the longbow man of the anaesthetic world. The rest of us preferred muskets.

~

I still ponder that Clydesdale anaesthetic but, when dealing with drugs—in animals as in humans—there is always the possibility of individual reactions.

I used to undergo regular three-monthly checks and operations for recurrent bladder cancers under general anaesthesia, so I found it particularly interesting to experience intravenous anaesthetics at first hand. When I met Joe, one of my anaesthetists on a social occasion, I informed him that he and his colleagues had knocked me out at least forty times in the previous twelve years. He riposted that at least they had brought me round forty times … "It's only when the two figures differ that we become really concerned."

My early experiences under Joe were with barbiturate anaesthetics, just as we had used on the colt. I am truly grateful that I avoided the roping down, strong assistants' era, the years when speed was merciful and lion-of-a-man Liston's ability to amputate a limb in half the time of other surgeons enabled him to inflict half the pain.

Each of Joe's anaesthetics followed the same pattern. I lie on the table. "All right John, slight scratch. Try to relax." Some slight scratch! The back of the hand is a sensitive area. He tapes the cannula in place as he chats about other things. Now he has a line into my vein. "OK, we're away. Breathe into this mask, John". An icy cold, intense ache snakes up the vein in my arm and a metallic, garlic taste fills my mouth. Very briefly, I appreciate why some dogs lick their lips just before they "go under" with a dose of barbiturate. That ache is intensifying, but the edge is falling off it … and I am falling off the edge. The chattering is fading ... Oh welcome oblivion! Nothing …

The awakening was somewhat less comfortable, depending on what the surgeon had been up to. But it was my personal experience of "going under" that gave me an insight into what I had been inflicting on my own long-suffering patients. It is not inconceivable that an icy ache searing your jugular vein could—if you were large and powerful, and just before the point when its effects claimed you—occasionally trigger a violent reaction; perhaps even impel you to rear up and brush aside your anaesthetist and surgeon before sweet oblivion overwhelmed you and you fell asleep.

Chapter Twenty-eight

Cancer: a Catalyst for Change

The future ain't what it used to be. – Yogi Berra

For much of my life, I wanted nothing more than to be a practising vet. Eventually I had succeeded in reaching the next rung, a shareholding in my own veterinary practice. The partnership was going well. Business, with all the new dairy farms setting up on Southland's rich soil, was booming. However, as with any expansion, cracks were starting to appear. Veterinary business was becoming a game of promotion and marketing enterprise and, with the enormous herds, some up to two thousand cows, it was increasingly a game of numbers. The work became less varied and more physically demanding. You could be pinned down for hours on one farm doing nothing but lame cows or pregnancy testing, or fertility checks. We had had such jobs on the large sheep farms, but they were carried out in a more convivial manner, at a gentler pace, with shepherds and other workers we had come to know well over the years. Even on the large sheep stations we were invited to the cookhouse for morning tea or lunch and treated royally.

In my opinion, the entrepreneurs driving the change to ever-larger dairy herds are strangling the spirit that so convinced me of the vitality of New Zealand agriculture. Leveraging on capital gain, they have become the new land barons, buying farm after farm. Some are solely investors with few ties to the land. As vets we were tending to deal more and more with disgruntled and exploited staff who, lacking job satisfaction, regularly moved on. It was becoming more difficult to establish trust and develop satisfactory working relationships in this environment.

It would be wrong to paint a totally negative picture. We still had a tremendous amount of work with sheep farmers and their dogs, and there were some motivated and considerate dairy farmers, but the more intensive dairying took over, the less it appealed to me. My mindset about being a practising vet, the only career I had ever considered desirable, was changing.

There were other factors in my change of heart. For several years I had been under treatment for recurring bladder cancer. On top of this, another seriously malignant form of cancer had erupted in my mouth. When I first felt the small pea-like lump catching on my tongue, and peered in the mirror to see what it was, I was horrified. It looked, to me, suspiciously like a squamous cell carcinoma (SCC). I had quite often seen similar growths in the mouths of dogs and cats. They were highly malignant and the prognosis was invariably grim, with the probability of euthanasia just round the corner. But, for myself, I thought it prudent to seek a second opinion.

Within weeks I was admitted to Dunedin hospital for removal of what had, indeed, been confirmed as a SCC, and a radical resection of the surrounding tissues inside my mouth. The surgeon also planned to remove the lymph nodes draining the area. This would involve delicately dissecting past the rich nerve supply to my left arm and he warned me that there was a chance that I would wake up to find it partially paralysed. What choice was there? I signed the consent form without hesitation.

It was with some relief that I awoke several hours later with nothing more than a numb cheek and a sore mouth. I was lucky, we had caught the tumour early and there was no evidence, from the lymph nodes they had analysed, that it had spread. But the immediate relief that I felt, and was reassured to see that Viv also felt—never having taken her affections for granted—was tempered by the warning from the surgeon as he took her aside and looked her in the eyes: "This is great news for you, but I have to be realistic. It may be seven months; it may be seven years, but it *will* be back."

It was certainly time for us to reassess our life plans. By this stage both Emily and Morwenna were undergoing tertiary education and well on the way to adult independence. The prime motivation for the working fifty year-old male is supposedly to grind out, during the years when he has the most earning potential, the wealth required to support him and his wife through the years of their retirement. Somehow it didn't seem so important any more. I wrote to my partners, advising them of my wish to drop off the after-hours roster. For much of my working life I had been on duty every third or fourth night. I proposed to trade a substantial cut in income for the opportunity to work a normal 8.30 am to 5.30 pm day. Generously, and in the same spirit they had carried me through frequent hospital absences, Giles and Sid (Daryl had by this stage retired to his farm) acceded to my request.

Soon after this I passed blood again. My bladder cancer had returned in a more invasive form and I realised that, once again, there was a reasonable chance that I would not be able to achieve all I had intended in this life.

~

251

It took two long months to recover from my bladder and prostate surgery. Two months of general listlessness, two months of pissing fish hooks, and at last I felt the stirrings of energy to get into the garden, to resume my work as a vet, perhaps even head into the mountains or the bush. But the histology report revealed that it was possible that not all the cancer had been removed. There was a thickening of the bladder wall on the CT scan. It was not something to ignore. The oncology specialist recommended a combined course of radiation and chemotherapy.

Even after eleven years of repeated monitoring and surgery for the occasional cancers thrown my way, this was the first time that Viv and I had had to face this dreaded prospect. Surgery had at times been scary, at times painful, but surgery is the clean solution if your cancer is in a suitable spot. As long as a tumour can be completely removed before it spreads and colonises other parts of your body, you have a great chance. Chemo- or radiotherapy suggests that the dogs of cancer have slipped the leash, and the dice are loaded that much more against you.

~

I found the waiting room at the oncology department of Dunedin Hospital a bit daunting, but I could not deny a certain Pepysian curiosity. It was new territory for me. How would I cope? Would I rise to the challenge serenely and with dignity? Thank goodness Viv was with me.

Other patients engaged in desultory conversations. We lounged in our practical grey gowns. There was occasional laughter, occasional exhibits of anxiety and things you'd rather not see or hear: "…I was OK last time until I started on chemo, and then it was like living with the worst case of flu you've ever had. After ten days I couldn't even be bothered to hold a conversation."

A sticky island of magazines occupied the centre of the room. In such situations men and women seek the non-challenging comfort of the women's weaklies, their limp pages pulped by the passage of a thousand sickly fingers. There were alternatives. Perhaps the pristine red covers of *The Fourth Labour Government: Radical Politics in New Zealand*? Who on earth would want to read that as their fate hung in the balance? Imagine the consternation: being called for therapy just as you were about to discover Geoffrey Palmer's views on constitutional proportionality.

Feeling disgustingly healthy, I set off for my first dose of radiation. The team of radiotherapists positioned me according to coordinates pre-determined by an earlier CT scan. The massive rotating head circled the hard bed on which I lay—no time for idle chatter as they retreated to the leaded-glass safety of their control room; they had another thirty patients to process that day. I had spent my whole working life juggling with lead aprons and gloves to protect myself from the cumulative effects of radiation, yet here I was, voluntarily consigning myself to another thirty-two repeats of a massive overdose. The radiographers were unconcerned by my questioning; it's mostly concentrated in a very small area. They warned me of tiredness, and other possible side-effects: diarrhoea, hair loss (oh well!), impotence (it won't happen to me!). And so with that age-old optimism, that enables soldiers to "go over the top", we accept our fates. Back then there was no choice. You got shot if you lingered. Death by cancer would be less humane.

When the buzzer sounded, did I really feel a wind of deadly beams pierce my flesh and shrivel my bladder? The mind plays games that scientific logic can't dispel. I chose to regard their risky passage favourably and willed them on. Blast away at the walls of my bladder! Eliminate every dividing cell!

So much for radiotherapy: chemotherapy is the one that really knocks you. Chemo damages all the cells in your body to some extent. Luckily, rapidly dividing cells, such as cancer cells, are the most susceptible.

Before starting, the nurse gave Viv and me a thorough pre-amble. Don't be alarmed when we approach you with full gown, mask and gloves. We don't know what the long-term effects of repeated exposure to even minute amounts of cisplatin could be to the nursing staff, so we can't afford to take risks. We ask you to consider all your body wastes as toxic. Flush the toilet twice after using it. Refrain from sexual intercourse for 48 hours, we can't even be sure that condoms are safe—so be careful! A fleeting thought— not even a careful act of unselfish conjugal charity with the protection of industrially reinforced gardening gloves? We grin at each other knowing, after thirty-three years of marriage, what each is thinking. Part of this is bravado: hair loss, diarrhoea and impotence feature as potential side-effects for chemo as well as radiotherapy. My immune system was going to be stuffed up. We were to avoid contact with sick people and pay strict attention to food hygiene. I was going to feel nauseous. Drugs would be given to alleviate the worst of these symptoms but some of these would also have side-effects.

Some of the same patients we had seen waiting for radiotherapy were already splayed out in reclining chairs in the chemo ward. Some dozed listlessly, but others, perhaps earlier in their courses, were more alert. They read, or chatted to friends and relatives. All the while they were hooked up to bags of fluid—often saline first, to lessen the noxious effects on the kidneys—then whatever chemical was being used for their type of cancer. By the end of the day, over seven litres of alien fluids had flushed through my veins, I'd wheeled my drip stand at least a dozen times into the toilet (my apologies, Nancy Mitford, chemotherapy is very non-U and they were not designated "lavatories" on this ward) and my kidneys would ache from their tough work-out. The mere thought of gardening gloves made me feel nauseous.

It started badly. The student nurse, poor girl, missed my vein a couple of times. Viv gripped my sweating palm in sympathy. Her support reassured me, but this was as much her ordeal as mine. Over the next few weeks she oversaw the gradual deterioration of my body into what we hoped would be a cancer-free zone. How far would I sink? Some of the patients—bald, jaundiced and enfeebled—bore witness to just how low you could be dragged. But it wouldn't happen to me of course, I just couldn't contemplate it.

We walked back to our motel. Many of the patients attending the oncology unit were outpatients, like us. With our home so far from the hospital we had few alternatives but to stay in a motel—subsidised accommodation. During the night I was up several times to eliminate fluid from my over-hydrated body. Being a law-abiding citizen I double flushed each time, as per instructions. Eventually it was too much for Viv: "Do you have to make that fiendish racket every time you get up? What about the poor people in the unit downstairs?" she hissed (in the nicest and most loving manner, of course).

"I was only obeying my nurse," I responded. "We wouldn't want to wake up in the morning and find the toilet bowl had been dissolved by my toxic emanations, now would we?"

From then on we flouted these particular rules in the interest of harmony in the motel community. If only the drunken louts in the street, the car door slammers and loud, late laughers had been as considerate. On St Patricks Day, in the student quarter of Dunedin, we cursed St Patrick and his drunken followers.

For the next few days I was conscious of what I dubbed "the pink smell"—something noxious pervading my deepest essence, so almost unnoticeable yet so very unpleasant. It reminded me of the slightly off-tainted pink juice from a long-thawed joint of beef. It was the faintest essence of nausea. After a while it did get to me. Its constancy wore me down. The gentle persistence of water torture is the closest parallel I can draw.

Sometime before my bladder cancer decided to spread its wings, a thoughtful friend lent me that book by Lance Armstrong (*It's Not About the Bike: My Journey Back to Life*). This mighty competitor, who has won the Tour de France a record seven times, bounced back from a serious bout with testicular cancer. Assertive from the beginning, he took control. He chose his treatment and his specialist. He came out on top. Is this the model to which cancer sufferers should aspire? Can cancer sufferers really fight their way out of it? If they then fail is it due to a lack of moral fibre?

Lance Armstrong chose a line that suited his character but, in my opinion, no one course is the right one. He was a statistic. A certain percentage of people with his type of cancer, given appropriate treatment, will recover and a certain number will die no matter what their attitude. The same applies to all those who disdain conventional medicine and place their lives in the hands of charlatans, radically change their diets, lifestyle, or religious beliefs. As to the appropriate attitude, there's a statistical bias. Not many people who fight and fail are in a position to record their demise.

Living in a small country, we haven't Lance Armstrong's luxury of choosing from such a large range of specialists. I prefer to assume that, in the main, New Zealand practitioners act in good faith and within professional guidelines.

Lance Armstrong got the right treatment and was lucky. I say this for all the people who lose their battle with cancer and feel guilty that their failure is for want of a fighting spirit, or for failing to top up with the latest panacea or diet fad that their nearest and dearest tried to foist on them.

At a more naive stage in our lives Viv and I had briefly flirted with the unpalatable Pritikin diet. However, Pritikin's basic premise—that if we restricted ourselves to vegetables only (ideally grass), we would massively extend our life-spans—didn't ring true for me, dealing as I was with farm animals. Ruminants, I had observed, were far from immortal: even without human intervention. Besides, Nathan Pritikin himself died of leukaemia—an inconvenience for his adherents and those who extolled his diet, which had been expressly promoted as a preventative for such embarrassments.

In the face of recurrent tumours, I tried to plot a course of serene acceptance, as far as possible. My fight was not to complain, nor to blame and become embittered. If, in the end, I was to win: so much the better. If I was to lose, I hoped to do so with dignity.

Week two followed the same format: daily radiotherapy, with Tuesday the dreaded chemo day. One afternoon I heard groaning from a changing cubicle. An old man was hunched over, a picture of misery. He didn't hear me asking if he was all right. I touched him on the shoulder, amazed at the soft flesh, and asked if he needed help. He looked up, and by way of explanation pointed to the urethral catheter snaking to a collecting bag on his leg.

"It's too painful to move now, thanks." he whispered, "I'll be all right after a short rest." His accent was heavily Central European: a refugee? A Second World War survivor? Very likely he would have known greater suffering in his past. To see him so sadly reduced towards the end of his life gave me pause for thought.

Over the years I could lay claim to more than a passing acquaintance with urethral catheters and the niggling pain and discomfort they cause. My depictions, earlier in this book, of Liston's tocolosi and Hollier's itinerarium, were not there by chance—such interferences, for obvious reasons, hold a special resonance for me. Likewise, I felt deep sympathy for my fellow sufferer. He didn't look like moving. He looked close to death. I informed the nurse and minutes later Viv saw him being slowly walked back to his ward. A few days later we saw him looking happier, the catheter removed. Where is the balance between pain and gain?

Amongst the reading matter I had been kindly lent for my medical internment was *Shackleton's Forgotten Heroes* (Lennard Bickel). This is a moving account of the team who lay food depots for Shackleton for the final leg of his attempt to walk across Antarctica. They accomplished the task heroically in conditions of great privation. Equipment was inadequate. Lives were lost in appallingly drawn-out circumstances. Men risked their lives for others. This was noble suffering for a cause, fruitless as it eventually proved: selfless suffering that inspires the human spirit.

In the cancer ward similar prolonged suffering, endured with great bravery, was part of everyday life. For the most part the pain and mental trauma were met with humour and good grace by patients and relatives alike. For many there was an end in sight: the hope that one day they would be restored to normal use and function, or perhaps the chance that a few weeks of suffering would buy a few months to support a loved one, or see a grandchild born. For others there seemed no prospect of restoration to a life of purpose and dignity.

I resolved that should the balance, in my case, tip this way, I would sooner float free, than drag on in the state of prolonged misery to which modern medicine and legal thinking—life at any cost—condemns many.

The pink tongue of nausea returned and gently lapped at every cell of my being. I developed angina: more tests and monitoring. I was in good hands. I could expect complications. The cisplatin was inhibiting DNA synthesis and denaturing the double helix in every cell of my body … but it hadn't dissolved the toilet bowl yet.

Deep down I felt optimism about the future. Viv squeezed my hand under the table. I had a lot to live for.

~

Week three, day five. The greeting card from a lovely dairy-farming couple said, "Hang in there, John". This

259

night I was doing just that. What positives can be taken from suffering? By enduring and overcoming such challenges, we have the chance to grow and become more appreciative, more feeling and more human. There seems little opportunity for most of us living our cocooned Western lives to come to terms with these things until it's too late. I wrestled with severe indigestion and, in attempting to sleep and take myself away from my discomfort, I repeated a mantra. Slow breaths: inhale… "as I suffer"… exhale… "so I grow". It seemed to help, and in the morning I was able to adjust my medication to alleviate this side-effect: one of many.

Gruelling days were to follow, but when I was halfway there and home for the weekend, I picked up a pen. Feeling listless and too debilitated to move from my chair, I lived for the moment, wrote of the moment… "I survey the sun-bathed garden through the window, much as childhood sicknesses encourage endless and detailed examination of ceiling cracks and wallpaper misalignments: endlessly, endlessly. But now I see the richly verdant bay tree, vigorous against the newly painted cream walls. It likes the position I gave it three years ago. Vibrant dark green leaves, in lanceolate perfection, alternate and dance up the stem, packed with the wonderful biological life-force of chlorophyll—the very essence of life on this precious planet.

I can only rejoice that I have been a part of this glorious, natural world."

~

Illness gives us time to reflect, time to sort out the past and plan the future. From now on my life would change. By happy chance, during the listless days that followed, I learned that my first book had been accepted for publication. Something I had been drawn to since childhood, but which had long lain dormant, seduced me as I wrote it: a love of words and the beauty of language. There was something else beyond vetting.

Chapter Twenty-nine

To Travel Hopefully

Little do ye know your own blessedness; for to travel hopefully is a better thing than to arrive, and the true success is to labour. Robert Louis Stevenson

The Victorians built solidly, and left a legacy of sturdy brick buildings the length and breadth of Britain. They placed an almost biblical emphasis on stable foundations. An amount of soil, at least equal to the estimated mass of the structure about to be constructed above the ground, was dug out for the perimeter foundations. It was then relatively easy to remove the surplus soil they enclosed and use this space. This neat solution explains why so many of these houses have capacious cellars. What a blessing these were for city-dwellers blitzed during the last war. People in cellars were protected from all but a direct hit.

On the other hand, these dank, dark, creepy cellars have inspired numerous horror stories, and hidden many unspeakable crimes. My experience of cellars led me to regard them as anything but places of safety. During my earliest teens—an age of imagination and uncertainty—I left my parents' coal cellar behind me for institutional life in the cellar of a large Victorian house. That cellar was the common room for the first-year boarders of my senior school.

First year boarders in School House were known as *trogs* for this very reason. The school laid a traditional emphasis on the classics so, naturally, this was an allusion to the Greek troglodytes: cave dwellers. The trogs' common room was no home away from home for the thirty or so boys who shared it. It was adjacent to a coke-fired boiler, which heated the whole building. Coke was tipped down a hatch into the coal cellar beside it and the surplus chunks spilled over into our locker room. The concrete floor was bare, patterned only by a filigree of cracks filled with coal-dust. From a romantic point of view, bathed in sepia tones, it could be almost have been described as Dickensian, and even adorned the lid of a chocolate box … and lo! … lift the lid and soft-centred cockroaches, black and crunchy, scuttle forth; as they did. The Reverend Black, he of the chasubled incantations in the school chapel, was our housemaster. When it came to the business of running a boarding establishment he was an eminently practical man.

As he had explained to parents aspiring to board their children, these cellar rooms were only a "temporary" arrangement, but the chronological timescale to which his use of this word applied was of biblical proportions. During my stay the décor and furnishings degraded further, into advanced dilapidation, as the boys afforded them the respect they deserved. The two settees moulted great clumps of horsehair. Their wheeled casters, continually abused in rough games by bored trogs, succumbed to the rutted floor. Eventually they subsided at uncertain angles, shabby relics slowly melding into the dim dinginess of their miserable surroundings.

For the most part the Reverend deigned not to visit his boys' common room, preferring to restrict himself to an elegantly furnished wing of the building, a world away from the nuisance of his charges. On Sunday mornings, after chapel, the first year boarders were herded into the large, sunlit study of this other world. There, the peace was palpable. After enduring days of echoing concrete, the opulent red carpets, curtains and wall hangings were a salve for the soul.

Occasionally the slight and beautiful Mrs Black could be glimpsed flitting down the hall, a memorable sight for us boarders; the only other woman in our lives was the grim, squat, and formidable Matron. However, we were not in the Reverend Black's study to ogle women, even if for some of us—yet to experience the perturbations of puberty—our longings were merely the innocent search for some mother substitute. Alas, it was made clear to us on our first herding into these Elysian out-of-bounds that our visits there were to be short and productive.

We were here expressly to write letters home, and to write letters home expressly …

The raised lectern looked strangely out of place in the Reverend's study; perhaps he used it to practice his sermons. He stood behind it and, looking down on us, drove his message into our lonely souls: "At this stage, boys, you are still adjusting to life away from home. No doubt many of you are feeling homesick. This is quite normal, and if you've got any spine, you will soon get over it. Remember, as you write, that this is also a wrench for your parents. It would be selfish, just because you are unhappy, to inflict your misery on them." He glared at one of his cowed charges, raised his voice a tone, and snapped out a withering: "What are you snivelling for Stewart? For goodness sake pull yourself together boy!" Calmly, he resumed—confidently in control. "I want to see you all fill at least one side of paper and I will see your efforts before you can go. Come up to my desk when you think you've finished. You have half an hour."

Could it have happened?… He shuffled his notes. A piece of paper fell off the lectern and drifted to the floor. "Well boy! What are you waiting for? Pick it up, there's a good fellow." The Reverend Black may not have heard of Kereopa's performance behind the lectern of the little church at Opotiki, but now I see it … Kereopa, on dropping Volkner's head … less messy… but the parallels were there.

But this did happen … Later, as we presented our letters to him, he dissected us in front of our peers: "This isn't good enough, Makliski. I've never seen such selfish rubbish in all my life! How upset do you think your parents are going to be if they think you're being picked on?"

And, quite audibly, in response to a whispered explanation, "Well if your parents have just got divorced, you might have to write a letter to each of them, but I can promise you, it's not going like that. Go away and rewrite it without that sentence. You have 10 minutes left."

With our letters duly written and censored by this man of God, we were dismissed to relax and celebrate the rest of our Sabbath with the horsehair sofas.

Steep gabled, gothic-windowed, grey slate roofed, grime-bricked, smoke-stacked, tile-floored edifices are you, the Victorian buildings of my youth. Your reverend caretaker occupied but a small part of the journey: a memorable traveller who crossed my path and served to alert me to other footpads I might meet. Within your confines the scales fell from my eyes. The sanctioned injustices were part of a living satire in which we all partook. They fed my sense of irony such that any foreboding I felt in your presence has now vanished.

As I revisit my schoolboy past, I can understand the shattering resonance I felt in later life when I first encountered *Gormenghast*, that brilliant fiction of

Mervyn Peake. The ghouls of my youth were reincarnated in the Gothic vastness of his fantastical creation. And when I had absorbed one of many sentences of consummate beauty, I left the final portion of his sinister world unread and unknown to me. I had tasted literary perfection:

Who are these dead – these victims of violence who no longer influence the tenor of Gormenghast save by deathless repercussion? For ripples are still widening in dark rings and a movement runs over the gooseflesh waters though the drowned stones lie still.

What could be more flawlessly realised for those who have gazed into the clear barrenness of a mountain tarn and seen, beneath the gooseflesh waters, "the drowned stones lie still"? I did not wish to disturb their pristine peace. Perhaps if I read through to the last sentence of *Gormenghast* the magic would evaporate: the stones rest dry and lifeless. Let them lie as they are for me: literary markers in pages of fluid prose. For that is the important lesson. If you enjoy the journey, sometimes you should make the effort not to finish, not to arrive. This is contrary to our modern, never ending quest to set goals and achieve them.

Likewise, I gaze west towards the mountains of Fiordland. What is important to me is that they are there, with *Gormenghast*, on the bookshelf of my mind. What I have seen of them I have loved—but I can never know all their secrets, the best parts could be, are likely to be, those I do not know. It is the unknown that feeds the imagination. It is reassuring to find that this is so, and that we can all use our powers of imagination to take us where we will. Perhaps a younger generation will yet find that it is possible to create a virtual world without the aid of a computer programme and come to realise that computers could eventually cripple our imaginative powers. As long as I live I will wish my eyes to sweep the crest of some distant mountain range and imagine the unvisited wilderness of gooseflesh tarns and drowned stones they protect. In this acquisitive world we must learn that in our lives we can't have everything. But if we have freedom of spirit: to imagine, to question, to explore; then we have everything we need. To travel hopefully is a better thing than to arrive. The journey is the reward.

My life as a vet, I now accept, was just one part of a journey. I feel immensely privileged to have reached my present milestone, never forgetting my constant and delightful travelling companion; without her the road would have been so much harder. My future lies ahead—paved with words, deliciously uncertain; but the drowned stones of history stretch behind, immutable and always there to haunt us.

About the author

I am an English trained (Liverpool University) veterinarian, recently retired. Apart from a brief stint in a dog and cat practice in Yorkshire, I have spent most of my working life in various parts of rural New Zealand working in mixed practice with sheep, deer, dairy and beef cattle, horses, working dogs and pets.

I have always been interested in writing and was the 'Vet Talk' columnist for *The Southland Times* for several years. My columns were usually of a quirky, or satirical nature—rather in the same style I have used for *A Wander in Vetland* and *Pizzles in Paradise*.

I have recently completed a novel, *She Bid Me Take Love Easy*, which is altogether another matter...

If you enjoyed this book, you might enjoy *Pizzles in Paradise*, another veterinary title by John Hicks. It is available as an ebook from Smashwords.com

Beaglehole, JC. *The Life of Captain James Cook.* Stanford University Press, California, 1974.

Bickle, Lennard. *Shackleton's Forgotten Men: the untold tragedy of the Endurance epic.* Thunder's Mouth Press. New York, 2001.

Bishop, WJ. *The Early History of Surgery.* Robert Hale Ltd. London, 1960.

Blood, D.C. and Henderson, J.A. *Veterinary Medicine.* 3rd edition Baillière, Tindall & Cassell. London, 1968.

Book of British Birds. Drive Publications Limited. 2nd Edition. London, 1974.

Brooker, SG, Cambie, RC and Cooper, RC. *New Zealand Medicinal Plants.* 3rd edition. Heinemann Publishers. Auckland, 1987.

Bryant, Arthur. *Samuel Pepys: The man in the making.* The Reprint Society Ltd. London, 1949.

Bryant, Arthur. *A History of Britain and the British People, Volume 1, Set in a Silver Sea.* Guild Publishing. London, 1984.

Bye, Ken. *Trial by Fire Trial by Water: History of Otautau.* Craig Printing Co. Ltd. Invercargill, 1988.

Cawthorne, Nigel. *The Curious Cures of Old England*. Piatkus Books Ltd. London, 2005.

Cooper, Marion & Johnson, Anthony. *Poisonous Plants in Britain and their effects on Animals and Man.* Her Majesty's Stationery Office, London, 1984.

Daiches, David. *A Critical History of English Literature*. Revised Edition. Mandarin Paperbacks. London 1994

Fraser, Antonia. *King Charles II*. Weidenfeld and Nicolson. London, 1979.

Geering, Lloyd. *Wrestling with God: the story of my life*. Bridget Williams Books in association with Craig Potton Publishing. Nelson, 2006.

Gordon, Richard. *The Sleep of Life*. Penguin Books Ltd. Harmondsworth, Essex, 1976.

Hall-Jones, John. *Fiordland Explored*. AH & AW Reed Ltd. Wellington, 1976.

Hall-Jones, John. *John Turnbull Thompson. The first Surveyor-General of New Zealand.* McIndoe, Dunedin, 1992.

Hicks, J D and Pauli, JV. *Chronic Udder Oedema: clinical aspects of the syndrome and its connection with hypomagnesaemia and anaemia*. New Zealand Veterinary Journal, 24 (10): 225-8, 1976.

King, Michael. *The Penguin History of New Zealand*. Penguin Books (NZ) Ltd. Auckland, 2003.

Kinloch, Terry. *Devils on Horses: in the words of the ANZACS in the Middle East 1916-19.* Exisle Publishing Limited. Auckland, 2007.

Laing, RM & Blackwell, EW. *Plants of New Zealand.* Whitcombe and Tombs Ltd. New Zealand, 1964.

Latham, Robert. *The Shorter Pepys.* edited by Unwin Hayman Ltd. London, 1990.

MacKay, Margaret Elizabeth. *Customers and Green Men.* Whitcombe and Tombs Ltd. Christchurch NZ, 1967.

Miller & Robertson. *Practical Animal Husbandry.* Oliver & Boyd Ltd. Edinburgh, 1959.

Milton, Giles. *White Gold: The Extraordinary Story of Thomas Pellow and North Africa's One Million European Slaves.* Hodder & Stoughton, London, 2004.

Mitford, Nancy. *The Sun King.* Hamish Hamilton Ltd. London, 1966.

Naphy, William G. *The Protestant Revolution.* BBC books, 2007.

Peake, Mervyn. *The Gormenghast Trilogy.* Mandarin Paperbacks, London, 1992.

Plato. *The Essential Plato.* Translated by Benjamin Jowett. The Softback Preview, 1999.

Porter, Roy. *The Greatest Benefit to Mankind: A Medical History of Humanity from Antiquity to the Present*. HarperCollinsPublishers Ltd. London, 1997.

Rice, Geoffrey W. *The Oxford History of New Zealand*. Second Edition. Oxford University Press. Auckland, 1992.

Sacks, Oliver. *An Anthropologist on Mars*. Picador. London, 1995.

Shrewsbury, JFD. *The Plague of the Philistines*. Victor Gollancz Ltd. London, 1964.

Sisson & Grossman. *Anatomy of the Domestic Animals*. Fourth Edition. WB Saunders & Co. Philadelphia, 1964.

Walker, Robin E. *Ars Veterinaria: The Veterinary Art from Antiquity to the End of the XIXth Century*. Schering-Plough Animal Health, Kenilworth, N.J., U.S.A. 1992.

Woodham-Smith, Cecil. *Florence Nightingale*. Constable & Co. Ltd, London, 1950.

###

Lightning Source UK Ltd.
Milton Keynes UK
UKOW04f0726301115

263800UK00001B/21/P